RICHARD L. HITTLEMAN

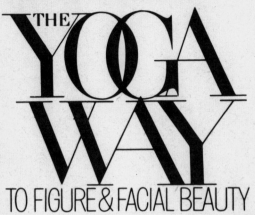

THE YOGA WAY

TO FIGURE & FACIAL BEAUTY

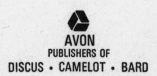

AVON
PUBLISHERS OF
DISCUS · CAMELOT · BARD

AVON BOOKS
A division of
The Hearst Corporation
959 Eighth Avenue
New York, New York 10019

First Avon Printing, February, 1970

For TONY, BRET, GREG, and CINDY

CONTENTS

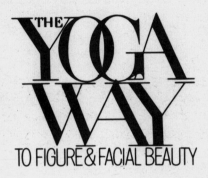

THE YOGA WAY
TO FIGURE & FACIAL BEAUTY

CHAPTER 1

NATURAL BEAUTY VS. UNNATURAL GLAMOUR

All of us want to be admired. Women, particularly, want to be admired for their physical appearance—their beauty. The need to love and be loved is basic in the human spirit, and since we are physical beings it is the physical presence of a woman that is usually first noticed by a man. Following that a woman's other attributes come into focus. But first we all notice the face, the figure, the walk, posture, hair—the component parts that go to make up the human animal.

So our multibillion-dollar glamour industry has contrived to capitalize upon the basic need of the female—to be admired, to be desired, to be loved. Look at the slogans and sales pitches with which we are all constantly besieged. Look at the myriad of products designed for the enhancement of the woman of today.

However, the true life of beauty is a natural one; it grows and is cultivated internally; without effort it is manifested externally. Physical beauty is an external expression of the spirit. Therefore, only a woman who has discovered her true nature, her "self," can be beautiful. Genuine beauty is all-encompassing and is present not only in physical appearance but in movement, voice, thought, and feeling. It is a quality that soothes and inspires all who come in contact with it. A woman is at peace with herself only to the extent that she develops her inner beauty. Because she has found herself she is able to give of her beauty—to her friends, family, and husband, and it is in this giving, and only in this giving, that true fulfillment is realized.

This natural beauty can be enhanced and externalized by natural methods—methods which are as old as recorded history but which only in recent years have been adopted by the inhabitants of the Western world.

Contrasted with natural beauty is unnatural glamour. The life of glamour is built upon deception. The glamour industry makes the woman a partner in its conspiracy by devising infinite forms of dishonesty and condoning her use of them. ("Look five pounds thinner without actually losing a pound." "He'll never know the real color of your hair.") Unnatural glamour is artificial and contrived. It consists of a series of imitations and exaggerations of genuine beauty. Whereas beauty is *internal*, unfolding from within, endlessly changing in color and hue, becoming ever more intense, glamour is *external* and its alterations must always be imitative, forcing the woman to continually change her costumes and masks like an actress in a play. Natural beauty is unified and whole; unnatural glamour is fragmented. In glamour there can be no true self-expression since it proposes that great numbers of women fashion themselves to conform to the current "looks" or styles that it manufactures and in so doing lose their identities. Glamour, therefore, implies conformity, but beauty is individual and distinctive. Each woman who has developed her inner nature is beautiful in her own unique way, and no one can ever truly look like her. There are potentially as many different types of beauty as there are women. This infinite variation is one of the profound fascinations of genuine beauty. The "look" of the beautiful woman is never out of style because, without effort and regardless of how she dresses or in what environment she functions, she is continually *making* the style—the style of her own unique beauty.

The Mark of a Beautiful Woman

A beautiful woman radiates from within; her complexion glows and her eyes shine. A glamorous woman imitates and exaggerates this phenomenon with cosmetics, mascara, and false lashes. The movements and gestures of a beautiful woman are poised and graceful; they flow with a natural rhythm. The glamorous woman attempts to copy these movements but she is never truly successful because they are not coming from her inner center. Rather, she is *imposing* them upon herself; they appear stilted and contrived. The body of a self-realized woman will be beautiful because she is deeply aware of her inner beauty, and this awareness manifests itself externally. The glamorous woman must conspire to mold or fake her measurements, changing them according to the proportions currently in vogue. The beautiful woman in her confidence dresses to please herself; the glamorous woman in her insecurity must dress for the approval of others. The beautiful woman, in contact with her true nature, is quiet. The glamorous woman, needing to perpetuate her ego, is ostentatious. The humility, compassion, and love of a beautiful woman are genuine, whereas these emotions are often forced by the glamorous woman, since she is unable truly to feel them. A beautiful woman is subtle and has a magical quality in her aura; the glamorous woman is overt and attempts to cultivate a mystique that usually turns out to be more embarrassing than mystical.

> A woman in search of glamour
>   can never be beautiful.
> A beautiful woman has no need for glamour.

The comparisons are endless since they occur at every turn of life, but the above may be sufficient to illustrate to the reflective reader that the tragedy of the woman living the life of glamour lies in the fact that she has sold herself short. She has compromised her self-identity, her self-expression. In choosing to be a copy rather than an original, she has sacrificed her own unique, individual beauty and with it her opportunity to attain fulfillment. The word "choosing" in the preceding sentence may be inappropriate, since most women are unaware that a *choice* exists. They are simply following the course of action dictated to them. Indeed, the idea of a choice would be the very last one that the glamour industry would want to have occur. That is why it has striven to make the words "beauty" and "glamour" interchangeable.

Choose a Life of Beauty

The first objective of this book is to convey to you that what the glamour sellers have sought to make one idea is actually two; to point up the distinctions between the two and make possible a choice; to have you carefully reflect as to how much of your life is now consumed in the endless pursuit of glamour; and to have you determine whether your happiness and fulfillment would not be increased were you to learn to relinquish this pursuit in favor of cultivating your natural, individual, unique beauty. The choice is actually between two very different ways of life, and your decision will depend largely on your present degree of unhappiness or disillusionment and on how strongly you are able to sense that real beauty lies within.

It is important to understand, beyond a doubt, that glamour is *external* in nature. That is, by adding to or imposing upon the woman various devices, clothes, cosmetics, jewelry, habits, mannerisms, services, possessions, etc., it proposes to make of her something she is not. Beauty on the contrary is *internal*. Every woman is born to be beautiful, and the seeds of beauty are always within her waiting to be cultivated. Rather than seeking to add to herself externally, the woman, in her quest for beauty, is led to discover and reveal more and more of her inner being, of her true nature, of her real self.

The male is very much to blame for the existing circumstances. He has been equally conditioned by the media to desire a female who displays the characteristics of glamour, and she, in turn, attempts to become what he expects. However, the woman who has seen through the glamour fraud is no longer preoccupied with this type of man. The development of her natural beauty will attract those with whom she can experience a much more profound relationship. Also, I know from many years of experience with my students that marriages can become infinitely more meaningful, since the woman is often able to elevate the relationship through her discovery of real values.

Now that we have seen how the life of beauty takes the form of a *continual inner unfoldment,* the second objective of this book is to present a method whereby this unfoldment may be initiated. The method offered is that of Yoga—an ancient and most remarkable science for awakening and developing a great force that lies within each of us. As this power is cultivated, indescribable positive changes occur and a woman begins to experience an unimagined beauty—not only on the physical level but in all aspects of her life.

CHAPTER 2

ABOUT YOGA

In the following pages you will be given approximately forty Yoga exercises. As you perform these you will be engaging in a wonderful adventure—that of discovering many things about yourself, your body, mind, and spirit. You will be joining many millions of people throughout the world who more and more are turning to this most ancient of all known self-improvement and self-discovery systems. Originating in that area of the world that is now India, the various systems of Yoga (there are a number of different schools of Yogic thought and practice) would seem to be as old as recorded history itself. As far back as we can delve into the Hindu legends and mythology we find mentions of "Yoga." The Yoga postures are described and depicted in the most ancient of scriptures. We can surmise through the study of these scriptures that the systems of Yoga were devised by men of great intellectual and spiritual stature in order to offer mankind a method of achieving health, beauty, and spiritual realization. The teachings of Yoga are not religious but rather universal in nature. They are applied by people throughout the world in every walk of life to attain many different goals.

The Yoga techniques of this book are primarily those of the physical or Hatha Yoga school and are offered here in the context of developing the natural beauty that is within every woman. Hatha Yoga is currently the most popular type of Yoga in the Western world. Through the efforts of numerous dedicated instructors and my Yoga for Health television programs, the great value of the Yoga exercises is becoming increasingly evident to Americans.

Although I often refer to the Yoga postures (Sanskrit: *āsanas*) as "exercises," they are not to be confused with calisthenics. The two are entirely different. You approach the Yoga practice in a calm, serene frame of mind as if preparing for a series of slow, graceful ballet movements. There is a minimum of jumping about, huffing, puffing, quickening of heartbeat, perspiration, and useless straining as is the case with most systems of calisthenics. From the Yoga movements we wish to *gain* vitality, energy, and life-force. We elevate our consciousness and become deeply aware of our beauty.

The following points are important. Read them and follow them carefully.

1. Perform the postures in a place of privacy where you will not be disturbed. Fresh air, even in cold weather, is necessary.
2. Your practice clothing should permit complete freedom of movement. A leotard is good. There should be nothing constricting on your body; glasses, jewelry, and watches should be removed.
3. Certain exercises require timing, so place a watch or clock where it can be easily seen.
4. You will need a mat or large towel on which to sit and lie. The color and design should be quiet and soothing. This should be used only for your Yoga practice.
5. At least ninety minutes should elapse after eating before you begin to practice.

In most of the Yoga postures the extreme positions are held static, without motion, while a few of the exercises are performed in continuous motion. Balance, gracefulness, and poise should be maintained at all times during practice, regardless of the type of movements being performed. All movements are done in a rhythmic fashion, and the necessary counting for these rhythms is given in the directions for each exercise.

Yoga Will Change Your Body

It is essential to understand from the very first day the *progressive* concept of Yoga practice. That is, you will be making major changes in your body. On certain days you will note excellent progress. On others there may be a temporary setback until your body adjusts to the new patterns. Some areas of the body will be stubborn and respond more slowly due to stiffness, neglect, etc. Don't be discouraged if you experience such a setback. Continue to practice easily and patiently, and in a day or two you will again be moving ahead.

We approach these exercises primarily from the standpoint of the development of beauty. However, each posture has many additional physical and mental benefits. These will become apparent as you progress.

Most likely you are particularly interested in one or two specific areas of your body—slimming your waist or developing your bust or preventing wrinkles from forming on your neck. But don't neglect the other exercises. You may emphasize certain of the postures in order to accomplish your purpose, but don't eliminate any of them because, at first, they may seem difficult.

The body is a whole organism, and each part has a relationship and interaction with the others. To develop a true natural beauty, to bring out the beauty that lies within you, it is important to do so with your whole body. All of the postures in this book can be done by anyone who will follow the directions.

Let us now begin. We shall apply the Yoga exercises to various areas of the body. As we do this we shall contrast the devices, gadgets, and products of unnatural glamour with the techniques utilized by Yoga students to develop their natural beauty.

CHAPTER 3

BEAUTY FOR THE HAIR

Unnatural *Glamour*	Natural *Beauty*
Curlers; straighteners; permanent waves; dryers; clips; pins; detergent shampoos; chemical colorings; sprays; lacquers.	Scalp exercises; correct brushing; sufficient exposure to air; organic hair products; proper diet.

Everything listed above under "Unnatural Glamour" destroys, to some degree, the natural beauty of the hair. By holding out the promise of "attractiveness" the advertisers have badgered, pressured, and duped women into enduring the innumerable tortures to which these products subject the hair and scalp. Surely, with even the slightest serious reflection you must reach the obvious conclusion that heat, chemicals, and styling gadgets can only damage the hair and suffocate the delicate follicles.

Is it really worth it? Is the appearance of your hair so vastly improved by the glamour devices as to warrant their continual and devoted use? We hardly think so. Your husband or male friends, in the final analysis, do not truly think so. When asked, men usually say they prefer the natural look.

The girls and women who today are allowing their hair to grow long, fall naturally, and who are caring for it with a minimum of chemical products and beauty salon "treatments" are in revolt against the contrived, artificial concept of beauty of the past several decades. Why not join this revolt—even if for a short time—and see what happens? If nothing else, think of the incredible time and expense that is required to pursue the glamour tortures; how much more constructively such money and time could be spent! But most important is the fact that once you revert to the natural care of your hair it will not only become more beautiful as the years pass (in contrast to looking more artificial and becoming increasingly difficult to care for) but you will feel *psychologically* less artificial and more natural. This is an extremely meaningful feeling, because it makes a profound difference in your entire appearance.

The natural care of the hair suggested for the Yoga student includes the following points:

1. Obtain a hairbrush with strong, natural bristles. Brush 100 strokes twice each day, morning and night.
2. Expose your hair to fresh air whenever possible. Wear a hat only for warmth or protection, not for fashion. *Your scalp needs to breathe.*
3. Shampoo your hair twice each week, three times if it is excessively oily. Use shampoos that contain as few harmful chemicals and detergents as possible. Castile soap is good. There are organic cosmetic shampoos composed of such ingredients as coconut and other natural oils. These are usually available at the finer cosmetic shops and health food stores. Give them a try. After washing, dry your hair in the sun whenever possible. It is better to dry with a towel than with an electric dryer.

4. Wear your hair closest to the way *it* wants to fall, not the style chosen for you by a salon stylist or this month's fashion magazine. Be true to yourself always and trust nature to know what is most beautiful for you.

5. Proper food is important. Your diet should consist of plenty of fresh fruits, vegetable salads, and adequate protein. A daily packet of gelatin mixed in fruit juice helps impart luster to the hair (as well as strength to the nails).

6. Practice the Yoga Scalp Exercise and Head Stand postures as detailed in the following pages. These exercises will improve the blood circulation in your scalp, thus lending vitality to your hair and helping to prevent thinning and falling.

7. If it is absolutely essential to tint or color your hair, choose a shade as close to your natural complexion as possible. If you are a natural brunette and you color your hair blond, you are in a foolish conflict with nature.

SCALP EXERCISE

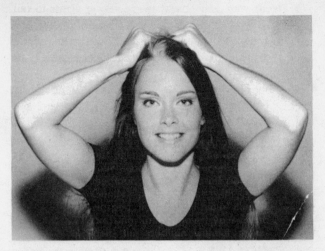

Fig. 1 Reach down deeply into the roots of your hair and firmly grasp as much hair as you can hold with both hands.

Fig. 2 Pull vigorously and *make your scalp move*, first forward, then backward as far as possible. Continue the movements rhythmically but not quickly. Perform twenty-five times.

Move your hands to the *top* of your scalp. Perform the identical movements twenty-five times.

Move your hands to the *back* of your scalp. Perform the identical movements twenty-five times.

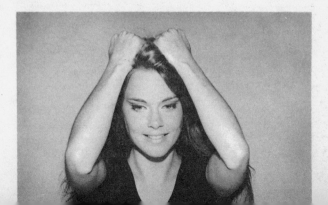

SCALP EXERCISE

• Do not slacken the firm grip on your hair while pulling.

        • Make certain that your *scalp* is moving, not just your arms.

• Don't be too gentle. It's supposed to hurt a little and leave your scalp stimulated and tingling. This is an especially good technique prior to retiring, after you have brushed your hair thoroughly.

Modified Head Stand—also good for the scalp—is described next under Beauty for the Face.

BEAUTY
FOR THE FACE

Unnatural *Glamour*	**Natural *Beauty***
An infinite number of cosmetics and appliances which make every conceivable promise from firming, tightening, smoothing, and otherwise rejuvenating to turning your face any size, shape, or combination of colors you desire.	Exercises to firm and improve blood circulation; correct care of the face, including natural cleansing; organic cosmetics, if necessary; sufficient exposure to air and sun; proper diet.

It is essential to understand that facial beauty is primarily an *internal* matter. There are no products that can be externally applied to *firm* the face. Firmness is the result of good muscle tone, and muscle is maintained by exercising the facial muscles. No machine or cosmetic can exercise your face. Only you can perform the necessary movements. To develop a naturally *smooth and healthy complexion* your blood circulation must be good. The blood brings nourishment and color into the facial areas and carries away waste matter, helping to prevent acne, blemishes, and wrinkles. You can create the illusion of a firm and healthy complexion with the use of putty substances, foundations, rouge, and colorings, but in the final analysis you are really deceiving and harming yourself. Remember that glamour deceives but beauty is genuine. The Yoga techniques offered here will provide the needed facial exercise.

Let us say just a few words regarding cosmetics. There is a vast number of products available, and these are designed by a multibillion-dollar industry to appeal to every conceivable facet of a woman's vanity. With few exceptions cosmetics (from the cheapest to the most ridiculously expensive) are composed of combinations of such "miracle" ingredients as animal fats, chemicals, detergents, waxes, extenders, fillers, and alcohol. (You might find it interesting to reflect on the fact that the jar or bottle in which your cosmetics are contained usually costs the cosmetic company several times that of the contents!) These products eventually extract their price from your skin in terms of drying, clogging pores, impaired circulation, discoloring, promoting allergies, and prematurely aging the skin. However, these things usually occur over a period of some years, so that by the time they actually become a serious problem the woman places the blame on "aging" and is forced into the position of having to search for some new "miracle" cosmetics to combat the effects of her previous "miracle" cosmetics.

This is not to say that aging has no effect on facial appearance. Of course it does. But to a natural, healthy skin and complexion the signs of the years are not a catastrophe. On the contrary, an older woman who understands and knows how to go along with the ways of nature retains her beauty for life. Indeed, she can often develop more real beauty in middle age than she had as a girl. The ludicrous and unhappy woman is the one who is determined to wage a continual battle with nature and resorts to every "beauty aid" she can find, as well as treatments, appliances, and even surgery in an attempt to disguise the fact that she is growing older. She may be in tune with the current glamour trends but is very much out of tune with herself, with nature, and with reality. Such falseness can lead only to continual unhappiness.

Natural Care for the Face

Regardless of your age you can turn now to the more natural care of your face and bring out the real beauty of *you* rather than become just another walking mask of the glamour industry. This natural care includes:

1. The Yoga exercises.
2. Continual and thorough cleansing of the face. Most soaps contain ingredients that dry and clog. There are, however, *organic* soaps as well as organic cosmetics. These are composed of natural ingredients such as vegetable oils, herbs, nuts, fruit extracts, milk, honey. If you feel you need to apply things to your face, we recommend that you try these natural products. Again, health food stores and certain cosmetic shops (you will have to search for them) carry the various lines.

The procedure which I suggest for facial cleansing before retiring is as follows: Wash thoroughly with a natural soap or organic cleanser (honey-almond cream, for example); rinse with warm water and follow with a cool rinse. Next apply an organic cream or lotion. Follow this with a warm cloth held over the face for about fifteen seconds, and repeat the cloth application several times. Then remove the cream completely with another cold rinse. Finish by applying an organic skin freshener.

The cosmetics in the above directions are necessary only if you feel the need for them.

3. Expose your face to fresh air and sunshine when you can. Do not be afraid of the elements; your skin needs them. Avoid suntan lotions with chemical tanning agents. No external substance is superior to sunlight in moderate amounts for supplying your face with nourishment. Avoid too long exposure to the sun.

4. Again, as with the hair, proper food is all-important in maintaining the health and vitality of your complexion. The skin thrives on natural foods such as raw fruits, vegetable salads, and complete proteins. Sugar products, candy, soft drinks, coffee, starches such as white bread, spaghetti, pizza, foods that have a high fat content, fried foods, and dishes that are highly spiced and seasoned are as poison to the complexion.

The question here is, Do you have the courage to be *you*—to allow your own unique, natural facial beauty to shine forth—or are you content to remain a puppet of the glamour industry?

MODIFIED HEAD STAND

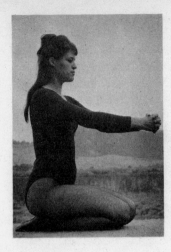

Fig. 3 Sit on your heels; interlace your fingers as illustrated.

Fig. 4 Slowly bend forward and lower your elbows, forearms, and hands to the floor, forming a triangle. Now rest your toes on the floor.

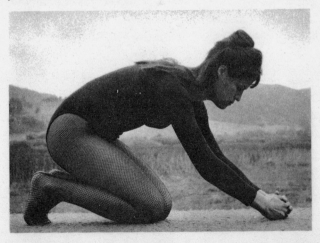

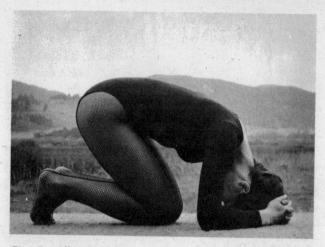

Fig. 5 Allow the front part of your scalp to touch the floor, with the back of your head resting against your clasped hands.

Fig. 6 Place your full weight on your forearms. Push up with your toes and slowly raise your entire body as illustrated.

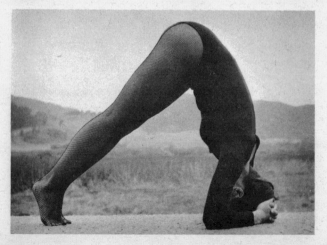

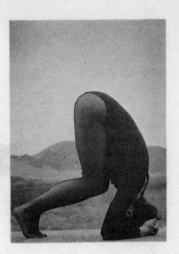

Fig. 7 Inch forward slowly with your toes until your knees are as close to your chest as possible. Keep your knees bent. This is the first position of the Head Stand. It is as far as we will go at present. Hold this position for thirty seconds (which you count to yourself).

Fig. 8 Lower your knees to the floor and move them away from your head. Remain in this position, relaxing your muscles as much as possible, for approximately 30 seconds.
Slowly raise your head and come into a seated posture.

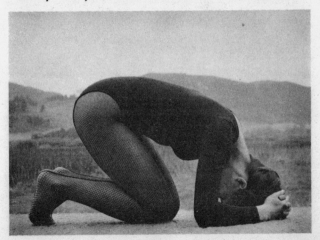

21

MODIFIED HEAD STAND

• This modified position of the Head Stand can be assumed by almost anyone with a little practice and is sufficient for many benefits to be experienced. More advanced positions will be suggested later, and you may wish to attempt them. Don't be frightened at this idea. You will have gained a great deal of balance and security before we actually try to go further with this ancient and invaluable posture.

• In addition to improving the condition of your face, scalp, and hair, this elementary position of the Head Stand, which gently brings extra blood into your head, can also help promote good vision, hearing, and breathing.

• Place a small pillow or folded towel beneath your head to remove the pressure from both the head and the neck. Direct contact between your head and the floor or carpet generally proves uncomfortable.

• During your first few attempts you may experience some discomfort as the blood flows more fully into your head. This feeling should disappear within about a week of practice and never return.

22

• Attempt *gradually* to increase the duration of holding in Fig. 7 from thirty seconds to two minutes. You can accomplish this by adding ten to twenty seconds for the holding period per week.

> • The correct position of Fig. 7 is extremely important if you hope to proceed subsequently to the Complete Head Stand. Note the straight position of the back and that the knees are brought in as close as possible toward the chest. They can be allowed to touch the chest. Later this position will enable you to shift your weight easily and maintain your balance as your feet leave the floor. However, under no circumstances should you attempt to raise your legs at this point.

• Never jump up suddenly from the Fig. 7 position without first resting for approximately thirty seconds as explained in the instructions. A sudden change can make you dizzy. Persons with high blood pressure or cardiac conditions should first receive permission from their physicians and always proceed cautiously.

> • Make certain that you carefully note wherever the word *"slowly"* appears in the directions. If you catch yourself moving quickly, slow it down. Remember, this slow-motion pace is necessary throughout all of the Yoga exercises. It will give you the sense of control and discipline that are vital factors in the development of beauty.

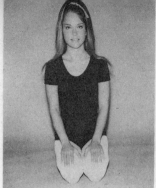

LION

Fig. 9 Sit on your heels. If this is uncomfortable sit in a simple cross-legged posture. Rest your hands on your knees. During a slow rhythmic count of five, perform the following movements:

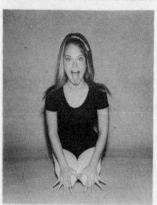

Fig. 10 Widen your eyes and keep them wide. Spread your fingers and hold them tensed. *Very slowly* extend your tongue as far out and down as it can go. These movements are completed during a count of five. Hold this very tensed position for a count of five.

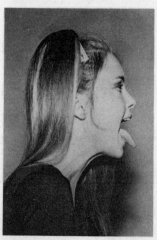

Fig. 11 A close-up. Note the extreme tension in the neck area.

Without pause begin the next count of five and perform the following movements: Very slowly withdraw your tongue; relax your eyes and fingers; settle slowly back into the position of Fig. 9.

Without pause begin the next count of five and repeat the movements of Fig. 10. Perform five to ten times.

LION

• These movements are performed within a rhythmic count of three groups of five. So begin the five count in your mind and keep it going steadily.

> • When you widen your eyes, attempt to bring into play all of the muscles surrounding them. This is good to help reduce crow's-feet and also reduce the tightness and tension that occur in this area. Make sure to keep your eyes wide during the movements of Fig. 10. The extreme spread of your fingers is good exercise for them.

• Your tongue must be extended *slowly* and then held as far out and down as possible. Don't slacken the tenseness until the five count is finished. If you do not feel a great tension in your neck and face muscles you are not putting in sufficent effort. (Study Fig. 11.)

> • By massaging the larynx, the Lion helps to maintain a nice tone in your voice and prevents it from becoming pinched and harsh. The movements also seem to soothe the throat, and we have found this to be excellent for speakers, smokers, and people with sore throats in general. Try it the next time your throat troubles you.

• During the hold of Fig. 10, certain areas of your face will have the blood drained from them. When you return to the position of Fig. 9 you will experience a warm glow in your face as the circulation increases. This exercise should leave your face and neck revitalized and toned.

> • Don't be reluctant to make the peculiar face required in Fig. 10. For the greatest benefit you must become ferocious. Think like a lion.

CHIN MOVEMENTS | *Important notes*

• Maintain an erect posture with the spine straight throughout these movements. Do not slump or allow the trunk to bend. Only the head is rolled backward.

> • In Fig. 13 make sure that the skin of the throat and chin becomes very taut.

CHIN MOVEMENTS

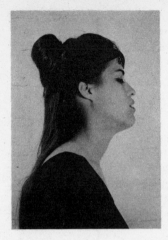

Fig. 12 In a comfortable seated posture, allow the jaw to slacken and go completely limp. The mouth is open.

Fig. 13 (Below) protrude your jaw and raise it very slowly until your bottom teeth are over the upper front teeth. Hold without movement for a count of five.

Relax and slowly lower your jaw. Without pause repeat. Perform ten times.

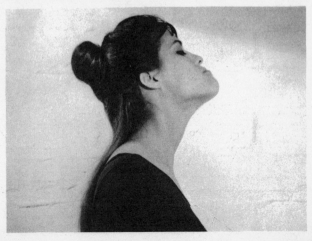

CHAPTER 5

BEAUTY FOR THE NECK

Unnatural *Glamour*	Natural *Beauty*
The use of various cosmetics in an attempt to smooth, firm, and disguise wrinkles.	Methodical exercises to keep the neck firm, graceful, and free of tension; additional exercises to maintain good blood circulation.

The beauty of the neck lies in its graceful lines and movement. A stiff or tense neck forces the head to move in an awkward manner and imparts a cramped appearance to the entire body. You probably will recall that on occasions when you have had a "stiff" neck you feel and look anything but beautiful.

As with the face, beauty for the neck is essentially a matter of performing certain methodical movements. Those that follow will remove and keep stiffness and tension from your neck, especially if practiced on a daily basis. These exercises will also help to impart a longer, more graceful appearance to your neck.

Other Yoga exercises such as the Lion, Chin Exercise, Head Stand, and Shoulder Stand help to firm by exercising the neck muscles and aid in preventing wrinkles by bringing an increased supply of blood into the neck area.

Use whatever cosmetics you feel are necessary at this point, but begin your Yoga neck movements without delay. Cosmetics cannot firm or rejuvenate. Exercise can.

HEAD ROLL

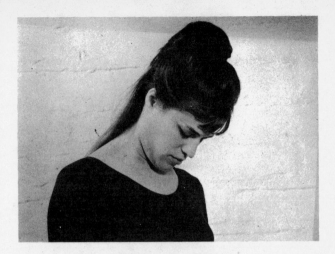

Fig. 14. In a comfortable seated posture close your eyes. Allow your head to come forward, and rest your chin against your chest if possible. Hold without motion for a count of ten.

Fig. 15 Very slowly roll your head to the extreme left position and hold without motion for a count of ten.

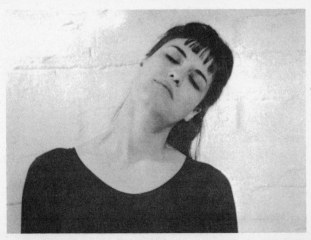

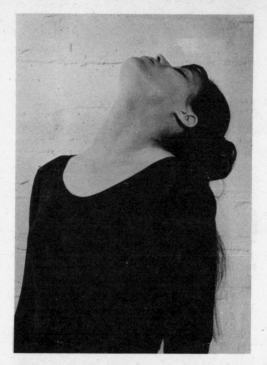

Fig. 16 Very slowly roll your head to the extreme backward position and hold without motion for a count of ten.

Very slowly roll your head to the extreme right position and hold without motion for a count of ten.

Very slowly roll your head to the front position so that your chin rests against your chest as in Fig. 14. Hold without motion for a count of ten.

Repeat the movements, but this time move *clockwise*, that is, begin the movements by rolling your head to the extreme *right* position. When these clockwise movements are completed, repeat the entire routine by rolling once more counterclockwise and once more clockwise.

HEAD ROLL

• It is essential to move in a slow-motion pace for this exercise. You have seen people trying to work out a stiff neck by turning, twisting, or jerking their heads quickly from side to side or up and down. They are seldom able to reach and work out the tight spots. Here we methodically massage and loosen, hence the reason for the slowness of movement and the all-important *holds* in the extreme positions. The more slowly you roll your head, the more you benefit.

• Make certain you are not just *turning* your head but that you are *rolling* into the extreme positions. There is an important difference between the two.

• With your eyes closed you can concentrate on the movements and try to feel your various neck muscles working out as you slowly roll from one position to another.

• Remember that only your head moves, not your trunk. Sit erect and don't let your body list to the sides or backward.

• These are also excellent movements to relieve tension and headaches. Try them next time before you take pills.

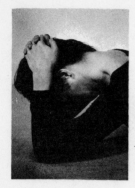

Fig. 17 Lie with your abdomen on the floor. Clasp your hands and rest them firmly on the back of your head. Lower your elbows to the floor. Keep your arms parallel. Gently push down with your clasped hands until your chin is pressing firmly against your chest. Hold this position without movement for a count of ten.

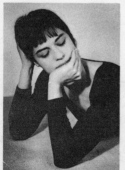

Fig. 18 Slowly raise your head and rest your chin in your *left* palm. Place your right hand firmly on the back of your head. Use your hands to turn your head slowly as far to the *left* as possible. Hold without motion for a count of five.

Next allow your head to turn slightly frontward for a moment and then *without pause* resume a firm grip with your hands and turn to the extreme left again. *Without pause* allow your head to turn slightly frontward for a moment and then turn to the extreme left once again. Repeat these *continuous* movements ten times.

Fig. 19 Do not move your arms. Turn your head so that your chin rests in your *right* palm and your left hand firmly grips the back of your head. Slowly turn your head as far to the *right* as possible. Hold for a count of five. Allow your head to turn slightly frontward for a moment and then without pause firmly turn again to the extreme right position. Repeat these continuous movements ten times.

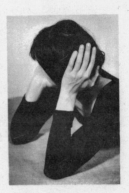

Rest your cheek on your mat and relax.

HEAD TWIST | *Important notes*

• This is a more intensive series of movements than in the previous Head Roll exercise. Here your hands are employed to turn your head quite a bit farther than is possible without their use and by so doing reach what may be sagging or unused muscles.

• In Fig. 19 you move in a *continuous* fashion. The objective here is to massage and loosen your neck by trying, in each of the five movements, to turn the head a fraction of an inch farther. So note carefully that although you are *holding* for a count of ten in Fig. 17, you are then moving *continuously* in the movements of Fig. 18.

• Do not make any sudden or erratic movements. If your neck is exceptionally stiff proceed cautiously.

> • Keep your arms parallel. If your elbows start to spread out you will not have sufficient height.

• You must keep a very secure grip on your head with your hands when turning to the extreme positions. Do not simply rest your hand on the back of your head, but hold it firmly.

> • Note the position of the fingers in the turning movements. Many students place them incorrectly. When you turn to the *left,* as in Fig. 18, your fingers are on your *left* cheek and on your *right* cheek in turning to the *right*.

• Close your eyes and enjoy the feeling of neck tension melting away.

CHAPTER 6

BEAUTY FOR THE BUST

Unnatural *Glamour*	Natural *Beauty*
Various apparel to achieve a desired size or shape; surgery.	Methodical exercise—in this case the Yoga postures—to develop the bust, maintain firmness and improve the contour, if possible.

The great emphasis placed by the glamour industry on the desirability of a particular bust size or shape has forced women to become more deceptive about this area of their bodies than any other. The fact that highly varying bust measurements can be simultaneously in vogue has led to certain ironic situations. It is, for example, amusing and at the same time sad to see large-busted women who decide that the "Twiggy" look is for them, or to find that the Playboy bunny has become the heroine for a small-busted girl. The various devices to which these females must resort in order to achieve the desired appearance is bizarre, humorous, harmful. Even surgery, a tragedy in my opinion, is not beyond the vain woman. And, of course, one cannot help but be most curious about the "moments of truth" which are certainly inevitable in love affairs. How is the deception explained to the startled male? Is he not somewhat suspicious of his lover's true nature after this disclosure?

Surely a woman who is intent upon being *herself* will not wish to deceive anyone, least of all herself, regarding her measurements. She will learn to appreciate her own particular structure, dress tastefully to accommodate her shape, exercise intelligently to develop her potential, and become beautiful by so doing.

It is impossible to state categorically that the Yoga exercises—or any system of exercises—will produce a desired effect on the bust. The factors involved include structure and glandular condition, and we cannot always predict with certainty how these will respond to the bust exercises. A great many women in our classes have been delighted with the development and improvement in contour that has occurred through the Yoga movements. Others have not experienced such dramatic results. However, there is no question of benefit, simply the degree of benefit.

The Importance of Posture

We must not forget the vital importance of good posture both for the beauty of the bust line and for the beauty and health of the body in general. A stooped posture in which the trunk slumps and the shoulders are rounded causes the bust to sag. This negates the entire attitude of beauty and vitality and causes a woman to appear and feel older than she is. Indeed, one of the surest signs of "aging" is the inability to sit, stand, and walk with the spine naturally erect and the shoulders back.

The posture problem usually lies in the back, spine,

and shoulders. (An excessively tight or ill-fitting brassiere can be a contributing factor.) The former two we will discuss under Beauty for the Back; the shoulder problem can be helped to a very great degree and often solved entirely with the four powerful Yoga exercises that follow. Each of these movements requires the shoulders to be brought up and back, and they are often locked in these positions for some seconds. Continuous repetition of these movements can gradually "fix" the shoulders in the correct posture. The improvement in the appearance of the bust as this occurs is often quite dramatic.

Remember that good posture cannot be forced. Glamour girls who attempt to appear "desirable" with a forced posture actually look ridiculous. To be truly beautiful a good posture must look and feel natural. The Yoga movements can help you to accomplish this.

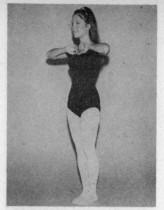

CHEST EXPANSION

Fig. 20 Stand erect with your feet close together and your arms at your sides. In a graceful dance-like motion raise your arms into the position illustrated.

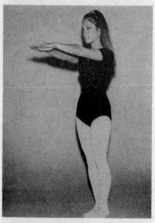

Fig. 21 Very slowly extend your arms until your elbows are straight. Hold your arms at chest level.

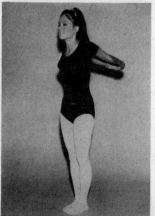

Fig. 22 Slowly bring your arms behind you as far as possible on shoulder level, then lower them slightly so that you can interlock your fingers.

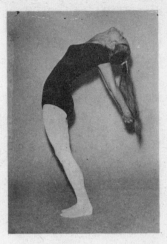

Fig. 23 Very gently bend backward an inch at a time and stop the moment you begin to feel the slightest strain. Look upward. Hold your extreme position without motion for a count of five. Keep your arms as high as possible behind you.

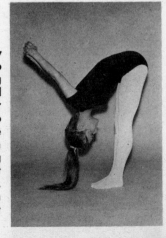

Fig. 24 Very slowly straighten up and begin to bend forward, bringing your clasped hands and straight arms as far over your back as possible. Do not bend your knees. Come as far forward as you can without strain, relaxing your neck muscles so that your head hangs limply. Hold your extreme position without motion for a count of ten.

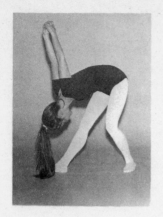

Fig. 25 Raise your trunk several inches so that you can move your right leg to the position illustrated. Twist your trunk to the right and bend forward once again, this time attempting to bring your forehead as far toward your right knee as possible. If you bend your left knee you can increase the forward movement. Hold your extreme position without motion for a count of ten.

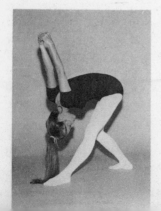

Fig. 26 Raise your trunk several inches so that you can draw your right leg in and extend your left leg to the side. Repeat the identical movements with your left leg and hold for a count of ten.

Very slowly straighten to the starting position of Fig. 20.

Repeat the entire routine.

CHEST EXPANSION

• In addition to aiding the development and firming of your bust this posture offers the following benefits: Your arms are strengthened and firmed through the movements of Figs. 22–26. Tension in your shoulders is also relieved through the same movements. The manner in which your shoulders are locked is excellent for improving posture.

• This exercise is unsurpassed for an immediate loosening of the entire spine. It will promote wonderful flexibility in the course of only a few days.

• The movements of Fig. 23 in which you bend backward are very powerful, consequently move cautiously. Remember to keep your arms straight and to look upward so that your head is back.

• In Fig. 24 your arms are brought far over your back to loosen your shoulders and your head hangs down to relax your neck. It is the holding of your extreme position without motion (regardless of how far down this may be) that will gradually work out each vertebra and allow your forehead to touch your knees. Do not be discouraged if you find your spine exceptionally stiff when you begin this exercise. This will be worked out.

41

• The movements of Figs. 25 and 26 will stretch the "ham string" muscles where people often experience stiffness and cramps.

• The Chest Expansion posture does not necessarily require exercise clothing and can be done at any time of the day when back, shoulder, or leg tension is a problem.

BUST EXERCISE

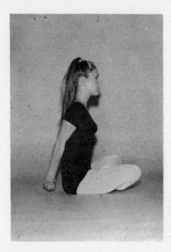

Fig. 27 Sit erect in a cross-legged posture. Reach behind you and interlace your fingers.

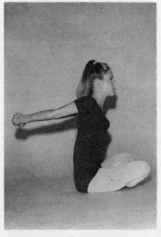

Fig. 28 Extend your arms and attempt to straighten your elbows. Very *slowly* raise your arms as high as possible. Look upward.

Hold without motion for a count of five.

Slowly lower your arms and relax. Repeat.

Perform the Bust Exercise ten times.

BUST EXERCISE

• This is a modification of the Chest Expansion exercise. Here you use only the first few movements to exercise intensely your pectoral muscles.

> • You will feel the firming and tightening of these muscles as you slowly raise your arms to the extreme position and hold.

• In Fig. 28 success in straightening your elbows will vary with the individual, being dependent on the structure of your arms. Make your best effort. Keep your spine straight throughout the movements. Slowness is essential.

> • This exercise can also be done in a straight-back chair to relieve the tightness and fatigue that result from writing, reading, typing, etc., at one's desk.

HAND CLASP

These movements should be done directly following the Bust Exercise. Remain seated. If your legs become uncomfortable in any of the seated exercises, stretch them straight out before you and massage your knees a moment, then come back into the cross-legged position.

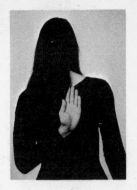

Fig. 29 Place your left hand against your back with the palm facing away from you as depicted.

Fig. 30 Reach over your shoulder with your right hand and attempt to clasp the fingers of your left hand. A few moments of struggle may be necessary to accomplish this. Sit erect. Now attempt to pull up gently with your right hand so that your left hand is raised slightly. *Without pause* pull down gently with your left hand so that your right hand is lowered slightly. *Without pause* repeat the up-and-down movements so that you do ten in all.

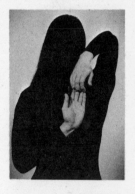

Unclasp your hands and relax your arms at your sides for a few moments.

Fig. 31 Place your right hand against your back, reach over and clasp your fingers with your left hand, and perform the identical up-and-down movements ten times.

Unclasp your hands and relax your arms at your sides.

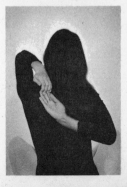

HAND CLASP

• Once again you are working with your pectoral muscles but in quite a different manner, as you will feel.

• If, in Fig. 30, you had to struggle to clasp your hands, you will find this will become easier each time you try. If, after a real effort, you are unable to clasp your hands, grasp the back of your leotard or exercise clothing with both hands and hold without motion for a count of ten. Then reverse your hands and hold as in Fig. 31. If you have patience you will find that you can soon make the hands meet. If your hands will not meet and you are just grasping your clothing, you will still benefit.

• You will find the movements easier on one side than the other. This is not important.

• There is an intense pulling and loosening of your shoulder muscles which will improve posture as well as relieve tension.

• Note that this is a *continuous motion* exercise. There are no holds.

BOW

Lie with your abdomen and cheek resting on the mat. Your arms are at your sides. Allow your body to go completely limp.

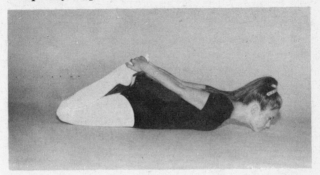

Fig. 32 (Above) Rest your chin on your mat. Bend your knees and bring your legs in so that you can reach back and hold your feet firmly. As in a movement of the previous exercise, you may have to struggle a few moments to execute the required hold.

Fig. 33 (Below) If you grasp your feet firmly you should be able to pull against them and very slowly and gently raise your trunk from the floor.

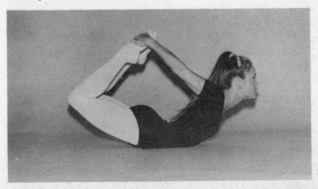

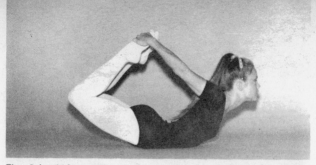

Fig. 34 (Above) The Bow posture is completed by raising your knees and thighs. Your head is held back. Note that the position of your body is that of the archer's bow. Hold as still as possible for a count of ten.

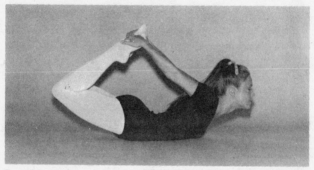

Fig. 35 (Above) Now attempt to "rock" to and fro on your abdomen, imitating a hobbyhorse. Holding your feet firmly, rock forward, bringing your chin as close to the floor as possible.

Fig. 36 (Below) Without pause rock backward, bringing your knees as close to the floor as possible. Without pause repeat the rocking movements five times.

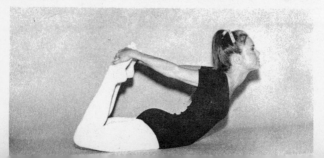

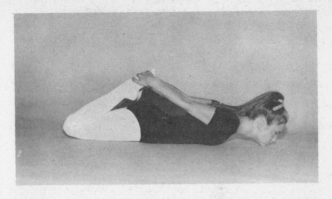

Fig. 37 To come out of the posture, first lower your knees to the floor. Do not release your feet. Next lower your chin to the floor.

Fig. 38 Only when your chin has touched the floor do you release your feet and lower them slowly to the floor. Rest your cheek on your mat and relax completely.

Perform the entire routine three times.

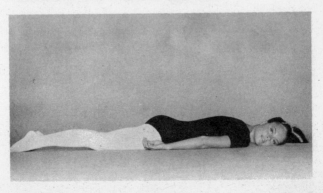

BOW

• This is an extremely powerful series
of movements for your bust, chest, back,
and spine.

> • In Fig. 32 you may have to struggle to
> grasp your feet. If this is the case, at-
> tempt to hold one foot first and then the
> other. Each time it will become easier.

• The movements of Figs. 33–36 are
highly strengthening and must be done
with caution. Never make any sudden
or erratic moves. You should practice to
achieve slowness and control.

> • It will be fairly easy to raise the trunk
> in Fig. 33. But raising both your knees
> and thighs in Fig. 34 is not easy and re-
> quires patience until the necessary mus-
> cles are developed. Continual practice
> will make this possible. If you *are* able
> to raise your legs without difficulty in
> Fig. 34, try *keeping your knees together*
> for added emphasis on the spine and
> bust.

• You must also develop control to perform the rocking movements of Figs.
35, 36 smoothly. In my classes I constantly caution students not to jerk or
fight during these movements. Try to
emulate the smooth motion of the hob-

byhorse. In this way you will never strain or "pull" anything. If you cannot raise your knees from the floor as instructed in Fig. 34 you will be unable to "rock." In this case simply hold your extreme position of Fig. 33 for a count of ten, keeping your head back. Then lower your chin to the floor (but continue to hold your feet) rest for a few moments, and repeat the raising of your trunk and the hold two more times. If you follow these directions you *will* eventually be able to raise your knees and later your thighs.

> • Note that this exercise combines a *hold* (Figs. 33, 34) with *continuous motion* (Figs. 35, 36).

BEAUTY
FOR THE ABDOMEN

Unnatural *Glamour*	**Natural** *Beauty*
Various apparel, girdles and contraptions to constrict the abdomen and disguise its size and shape; massages and appliances to reduce flabbiness.	Proper diet; Yoga exercises that concentrate on strengthening and toning specific areas of the abdomen not reached through ordinary exercise.

We will discuss the over-all problem of the waistline under that heading. Here, let us concentrate solely on your abdominal area.

From the glamour viewpoint the abdominal line must be held at any cost. It seems less important to cope with the source of the problem (overeating, insufficient exercise, loss of muscle tone) than to disguise the various bulges. The measures taken to implement this "holding" action have probably resulted in more discomfort to the human body than anything since the armor worn by the crusaders. As one examines the various garments of tortuous underclothing in which the glamour-conscious woman attempts to contain her expanding mid-section, one can only ask incredulously, "What price glory?"

An inescapable fact is that the stomach is located in

the abdomen and that the abdominal structure permits very great expansion to occur. The more one overeats and bloats the stomach, the larger the area becomes. This has an obvious negative effect on health as well as beauty. The longer the abdominal area remains overexpanded, the more the chance that the abdominal wall will lose its tone. When this wall is weakened, the organs and glands that it supports can begin to drop—a most unsightly and unhealthy situation. When the woman then resorts to squeezing the abdominal area ruthlessly with restrictive girdles, and other artificial devices, the problem is not solved but actually compounded. Therefore, the first rule of abdominal health and beauty is not to allow the abdomen to overexpand; one must not overeat.

Next, we can maintain the tone of the abdominal muscles, almost regardless of age, through the Yoga movements that follow. The Abdominal Lift movements are unique in that they actually require the abdomen itself to be moved. (Most systems of exercise attempt to work on the abdomen through trunk and leg movements only.) The Locust posture is a marvelous exercise to firm and strengthen the lower abdomen and promote the health of the reproductive system. Finally the Slow-Motion Firming is extremely effective because of the pace and rhythm in which the movements are performed. Remember that massages and appliances, even if successful in rubbing away an inch or two, are at best temporary expedients. For genuine tone and strength you must exercise properly.

We offer the suggestion that you gradually attempt to discard apparel that confines the abdomen and allow yourself as much freedom and breathing space as possible.

ABDOMINAL LIFT
(Standing)

Read the directions through completely several times and study the photographs before you begin this exercise. Stand with your heels together and arms at sides.

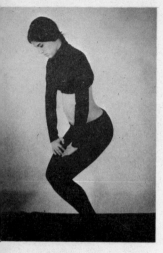

Fig. 39 Bend your knees slightly outward. Place your hands firmly on your thighs, all fingers pointing inward (including the thumb). Relax the abdomen.

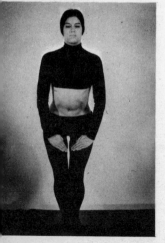

Figs. 40, 41 Now raise your abdomen. To accomplish this raising or "sucking in" of the abdomen it is necessary to do the movements with *the breath held out of your lungs.* You cannot lift your abdomen as illustrated unless the lungs are empty. Therefore exhale very deeply so that all the air is forced out and then use the abdominal muscles forcefully to contract and lift in that area. At this point in the exercise exhale as deeply as possible and empty the lungs. *With your breath held out*, work the abdominal muscles and attempt to contract and raise your abdomen. Hold this lift for a count of three.

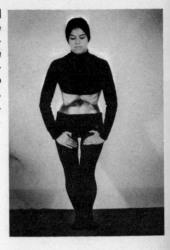

Fig. 42 With your breath still held out, attempt to *snap* your abdomen out. Do not allow it simply to relax and fall back into its natural position but use your muscles forcefully to shoot or snap it out. *Keep your breath out*. Without pause repeat these lifting and snapping out movements and do as many as you can *with your breath held out*.

Throughout these movements keep your spine erect; do not bend forward. Slowly straighten to the upright position and inhale deeply several times. Try not to fidget or become restless; simply stand easily and breathe deeply.

Return to the position of Fig. 39, exhale deeply, and repeat the routine, doing as many movements as you can *with your breath held out*.

Perform five rounds in all.

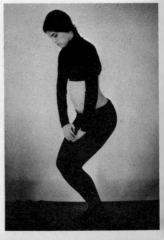

• In the beginning many students are able only to pull the abdomen in slightly without actually contracting and raising as fully as shown in Figs. 40 and 41. This is perfectly all right. Benefits will be quickly experienced from just a slight contraction. By continuing to practice you will catch on to the knack of deep contraction and raising. It is a matter of repetition.

> • Remember that the whole trick lies in preventing any air from entering your lungs until you straighten up and inhale. The emptier the lungs, the easier it is to raise. Therefore once you have exhaled as deeply as possible close your throat and keep it locked tightly.

• In Fig. 40 it is helpful to push your hands down hard on your thighs as you contract.

> • Students perform anywhere from one to twenty lifting and snapping-out movements to each exhalation. Naturally the number will increase with practice. A steady in-and-out rhythm is important for the movements, not speed.

• The snapping out of the abdomen in Fig. 42 aids in firming and improving muscle tone. Needless to say, your stomach should be empty when practicing this exercise.

ABDOMINAL LIFT
(All-Fours Position)

These movements follow those of the previous abdominal exercise.

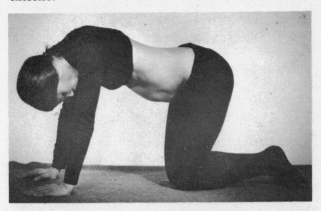

Fig. 43A (Above) Place your palms and knees on the mat. Allow your legs to touch and have your hands parallel on a line with your knees. Lower your head.

Fig. 43B (Below) Perform the identical abdominal movements as in Figs. 40 and 41. Exhale deeply, push down hard with your palms, and do as many lifts as possible. Inhale deeply several times and repeat.

Perform five rounds.

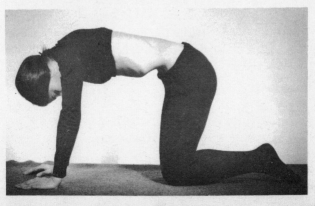

ABDOMINAL LIFT
(All-Fours Position)

• Here we work to firm the abdominal area with the body in a different position. This All-Fours posture will actually prove easier because your hands are supported by the floor.

• This is also an excellent exercise to practice after childbirth. Correct functioning of your various organs and glands is promoted by these movements.

ABDOMINAL LIFT
(Seated)

For the third Abdominal Lift position we take a cross-legged posture. If the posture illustrated is difficult for you, just crossing your ankles will be adequate at first. These movements follow those of the previous exercise.

Fig. 44 With your hands braced firmly against your knees, exhale deeply and perform the lifts exactly as in the two previous exercises.

Do five rounds.

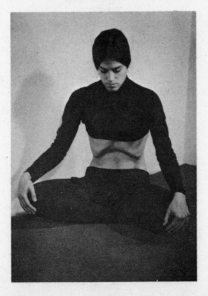

ABDOMINAL LIFT
(Seated)

• In addition to the firming and strengthening actions there are other important effects of the Abdominal Lift exercises. In these you can feel how the Yoga exercises work *internally*. The stomach, liver, gall bladder, pancreas, kidneys, intestines, colon, and peristaltic action are stimulated.

• The internal stimulation is particularly effective if the juice of half a lemon is squeezed into approximately four ounces of cool water and taken five to ten minutes before the Abdominal Lift exercises are practiced.

• Perform the three Abdominal Lift exercises as a routine, each position following the previous one with only a slight pause. You will experience noticeable results within a matter of days.

LOCUST

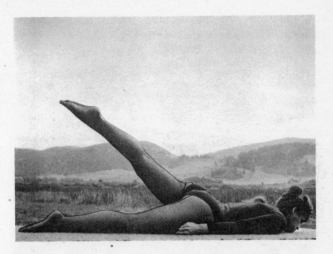

Fig. 45 Your abdomen and chin rest on the mat. Make fists of your hands and place them at your sides, thumbs down. Slowly raise your left leg as high as possible—pushing down hard with your fists will help. Hold for a count of five. Slowly lower your left leg to the floor and then slowly raise your right leg as high as possible. Hold for a count of five and slowly lower. The slower these movements are done, the greater the benefit experienced. Alternate the raising of your left and right legs and perform three times.

Now we will want to raise both legs. The working of the muscles required to do this will firm and tighten not only the lower abdomen but the buttocks and legs as well. Therefore you must make every effort to exercise these muscles regardless of how difficult it may be for you to raise both legs in the beginning.

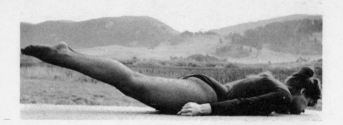

Fig. 46 (Above) Keep your chin on the floor during the following movements. Push down hard with your fists. Inhale deeply through your nose and retain your breath. Try to raise both legs; lift as high as possible without bending your knees. Continue to retain the breath. Hold whatever position you attain for a count of five. Slowly lower your legs to the floor, simultaneously exhaling deeply and with control through your nose (don't allow the air to rush out). When your legs touch, rest your cheek on the mat and relax completely until you get your second wind. Then turn your chin to rest on the mat and repeat.

Perform three times.

Fig. 47 (Below) A more advanced position, which is attained gradually with practice. The body resembles the locust or grasshopper.

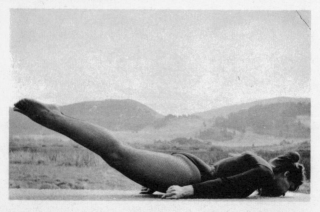

LOCUST

• In the case of most students the muscles required to lift the legs have grown weak from lack of proper exercise. Thus, in the beginning, both legs can be raised only a few inches. As soon as these muscles begin to strengthen, the legs can be raised increasingly higher. However, the distance the legs are lifted is not so important as is the effort involved.

• In this exercise the firming and strengthening occur in the lower abdomen, thighs, buttocks, wrists, and arms. In addition the Yogis state that the Locust movements stimulate the reproductive organs and glands.

• In Fig. 45 rest your head more on the ball of your chin than on its point for stronger support.

• In Fig. 46 the inhalation and retention of breath builds the chest for better support during the raising of the legs.

• When your legs are being raised, try to keep them as close together as possible. This places more emphasis on the abdomen and buttocks.

• The lowering movements of Fig. 46 must be done with control. Do not "collapse" and let your legs fall to the floor; lower them slowly. The same is true for your breath, which should be exhaled slowly and always through the nose.

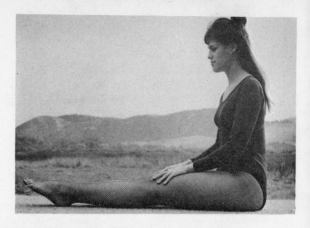

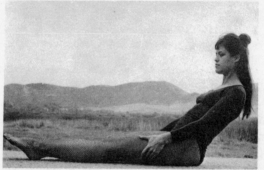

Fig. 48 (Top) Sit with your spine erect, legs together, and hands on knees.

Fig. 49 (Above) Grip the sides of your legs, bend backward, and attempt to lower your trunk to the floor during a slow count of five.

Fig. 50 (Right) When your back rests on the floor, begin the next count of five and raise your legs stiffly and slowly to the position illustrated. Keep your knees straight. Without pause lower your legs to the floor in a count of five.

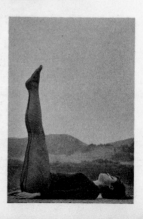

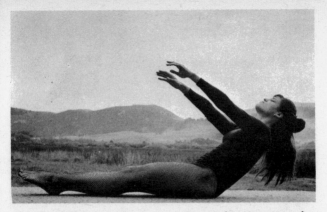

Fig. 51 Begin the next count of five and attempt to raise your trunk to an upright position. Try not to use your hands.

Fig. 52 During the next count of five bend forward slowly and grip your calves or ankles so that you can gently pull your trunk down. Time your movements so that your head reaches the farthermost point forward and down at the number "five."

During the next count of five very slowly straighten to the upright position of Fig. 48.

Begin the next group of five and repeat the entire routine.

Perform five times.

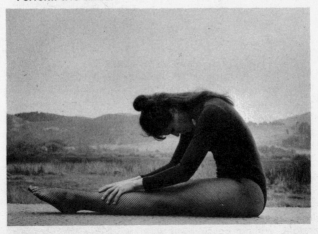

SLOW-MOTION FIRMING

• You will immediately feel the firming qualities of this routine. The movements are performed in continuous slow motion during the rhythmic counting of six groups of five. Keep the counting steady and make your body movements conform strictly to the "five" beat.

> • If you are unable either to lie down or sit up without the aid of your hands, then use them (actually you will be using your arms or elbows) until you have developed the necessary muscles.

• When you come forward in Fig. 52, bend your elbows outward and drop your head down so that you can allow your spine to experience an intensive stretch.

BEAUTY
FOR THE BACK

Unnatural *Glamour*	Natural *Beauty*
Massages, appliances, and various calisthenics to "spot" reduce and firm.	An intensive series of Yoga back exercises to streamline, firm, develop suppleness and flexibility, improve posture, help prevent joint and muscle disease, and relieve tension.

          The two necessary qualities for natural beauty of the back are firmness and suppleness. We assume that weight will be normalized through the use of our over-all Yoga program, that is, by performing the complete plan of exercises. Therefore we will not discuss excess weight in the back area as a separate problem. In Yoga it is not practical to "spot" reduce. We prefer to work on the metabolism as a whole, which will then conform with nature's plan for the individual organism. However, even though one is not necessarily overweight, it is possible to become flabby in any area of the body. The four intensive exercises that follow will firm your entire back as much as anything that can be done.

The importance of the second characteristic, suppleness, is usually not consciously considered. And yet suppleness and flexibility lend an indescribable beauty to the form and movement of the body, as we can readily see in the professional dancer. A stiff, tight, or tense body can be painted and clothed glamorously but it cannot be beautiful. Stiffness and rigidity are synonymous with aging and poor health; they detract from the free, graceful movements that the eye associates with true femininity. Also, since health and beauty are closely interwoven, it follows that diseases such as arthritis and bursitis, which stiffen the joints and cause such great discomfort, will make graceful movement almost impossible. From many years of experience it is my belief that the thorough, methodical movements of the Yoga exercises that manipulate the joints can help to prevent these diseases and keep the limbs and spine flexible regardless of age. The more your vertebrae stiffen, the older you are going to look and feel. A woman with a stiff spine can appear old at thirty. That is why the Yogis say, "You are as young as your spine is flexible."

No woman can be beautiful when she is in pain. You cannot look beautiful if you don't feel beautiful or if discomfort is written on your face. Back pain, particularly in the lower back (lumbar), is one of the major complaints of American women and often forces them to assume awkward, tense positions of the trunk. The Yoga back and spine postures have brought more natural, permanent relief for this lower back affliction than any other method of exercise. (It is quite possible that most systems of calisthenics tend to complicate back pains and strains.) As the spine is exercised and the various types of back discomfort are relieved, posture is often greatly improved. In passing we should also note that a straight spine and good posture help to promote alertness and clarity of mind.

The problem of tension, which can occur at any time to anyone and last for minutes, hours, or days, is also, from the Yogic viewpoint, a matter of tightness or "squeezing" that occurs at the point of tension. A body that is supple and flexible can minimize tension. The next time you experience a tenseness in your back, perform the following four Yoga exercises as soon as possible and you may experience wonderful, natural relief.

To maintain smoothness on the skin of the back an organic cosmetic can be used.

COBRA

The objective of this series of movements is to raise and lower the trunk in such a manner that *each vertebra, in turn, is exercised.*

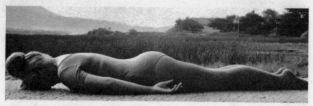

Fig. 53 (Above) Rest your forehead on the mat; place your arms at your sides and allow your body to go limp.

Fig. 54 (Below) Very slowly raise only your head, bending it far back. Without the use of your hands, lift your trunk as far from the floor as possible. Make your back muscles work.

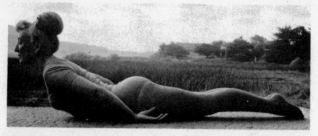

Fig. 55 (Below) When you can lift no farther, hold your trunk in the raised position and bring your hands in gracefully (as in a swimming motion). Place them in line with your shoulders, making certain that your fingers are in the position depicted.

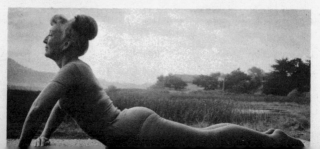

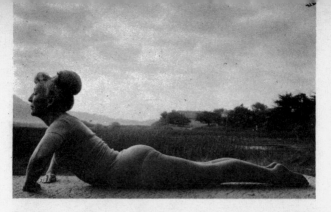

Fig. 56 Continue to raise the trunk *as slowly as possible*, using your hands for support. Your head should tilt backward and your spine is always curved. Do not straighten or stiffen your back.

Fig. 57 The final position with the elbows straight, head and spine in an extreme arch, and your legs relaxed. Hold for a count of ten. When the count is completed, bend your elbows slightly so that your trunk is lowered a short distance, then push back up slowly to the extreme position. Repeat these up-and-down movements very slowly so that you perform them five times for a complete loosening of your lower spine (the lumbar area). Then return to the extreme arched position.

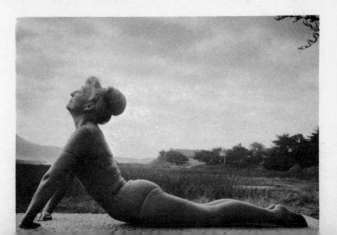

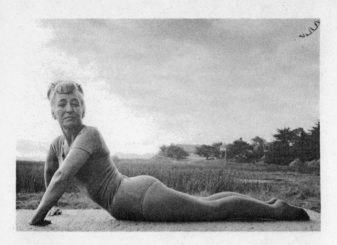

Fig. 58 Now bend *only your right elbow* slightly so that you can twist your trunk as illustrated and attempt to see your left heel. Hold for a count of five. Then return to the extreme arched position of Fig. 57.

Fig. 59 Now bend *only your left elbow* slightly and perform the identical movements by twisting to the right and attempting to see your right heel. Hold for a count of five. Return to the extreme arched position of Fig. 57.

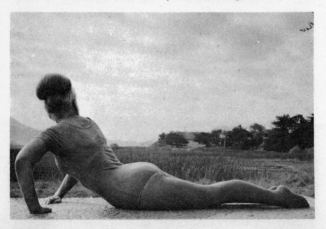

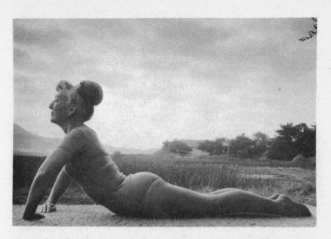

Fig. 60 Keep your spine arched and slowly lower your trunk halfway to the floor.

Fig. 61 Bring your arms to your sides so that your back muscles must once again support your trunk. Continue to lower until your forehead touches the mat. Rest your cheek on the mat and relax.

Perform the complete Cobra routine twice.

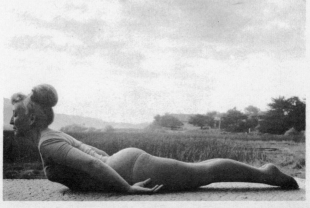

COBRA

• There is nothing comparable to the Cobra for relieving tension throughout the back and spine and for firming the lower back, which so often becomes flabby.

• Keep your head continually tilted backward.

• Your spine is continually arched, never straightened.

• Make certain the hand and finger position of Fig. 55 is correct.

• Keep your legs relaxed; they have a tendency to become tense.

• In the beginning days of practice raise your trunk to whatever extreme position is comfortable. Your elbows need not be straight (Fig. 57). As you progress you will be able to attain the position depicted and resemble a Cobra snake.

• Slow-motion movement is all-important in this exercise. The slower the movement, the more tension relieved and the more firming that occurs. Think of the entire Cobra routine as a series of ballet movements.

• The Cobra will also impart a wonderful flexibility to your spine. It helps to separate the vertebrae and has been most helpful in many types of back ailments. The more flexible your spine, the more youthful you're going to look and feel.

BACK STRETCH

Sit on the mat and extend your legs with knees and feet together. Straighten your spine, rest your hands on your thighs, and relax a moment.

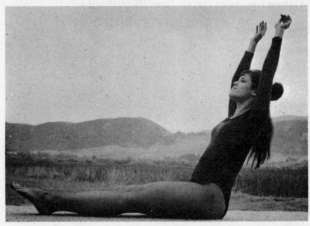

Fig. 62 In a slow, graceful movement raise your arms and bring them overhead as illustrated. Bend backward a short distance to help firm the abdomen.

Fig. 63 Execute a slow-motion dive forward.

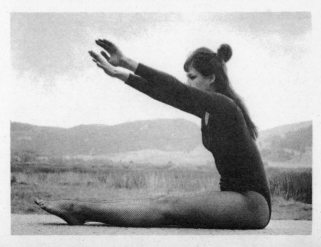

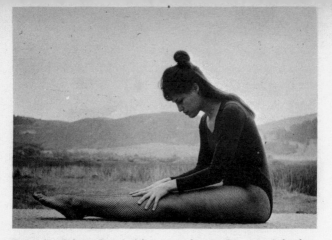

Fig. 64 Take a firm hold on your knees. Do not go farther than your knees.

Fig. 65 Pull against your knees, bend your elbows outward, and gently draw your trunk down, aiming your forehead toward your knees. Pull down as far as you can without strain and hold *without moving* for a count of five. Do not bend your knees. When the count is completed, continue to hold your knees firmly but straighten your trunk an inch or two. Note—an inch or two only. Do not straighten all the way up. Now once again pull your trunk down toward your knees, and when you have gone as far down as possible, *without pause* straighten your trunk an inch or two. Without pause, pull down again. Repeat these short up-and-down movements so that you do five in all. Thus we hold the first stretch for a count of five, but then do five of the up-and-down movements *without pause*.

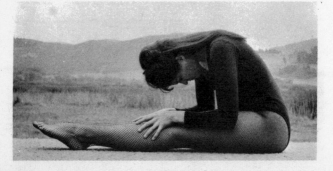

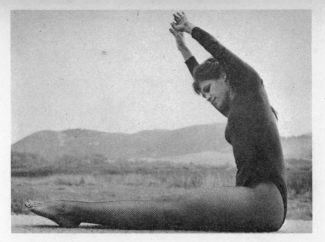

Fig. 66 Slowly straighten up, and as you do so bring your arms overhead once again. Slowly begin to dive forward as before, this time gently rocking or swaying to and fro as you come down. (This helps to loosen the spine.)

Fig. 67 Now attempt to take a firm hold on your calves. Do not go farther than your calves. Pull against your calves, bend your elbows, and gently draw your trunk down, again aiming your forehead toward your knees. Do not bend your knees. Hold your extreme position for a count of five.

Continue to hold the calves firmly, but raise the trunk an inch or two. Without pause, pull down again and perform the up-and-down movements five times, slowly as before. If you are unable to reach your calves, simply hold the knees as before and repeat the identical movements.

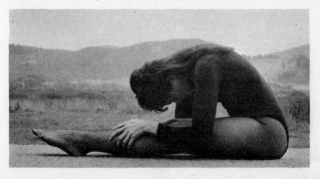

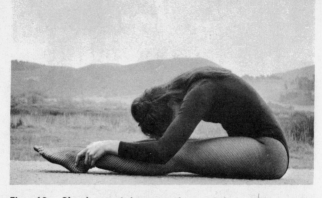

Fig. 68 Slowly straighten to the upright position, raise your arms overhead, perform the rocking movements again, and this time attempt to hold the ankles. Draw down, hold for five, perform the to-and-fro movements five times. If you cannot reach your ankles, simply hold your knees or calves and repeat the identical movements.

Fig. 69 Slowly straighten up and once again perform the rocking movements, this time reaching very far forward and attempting to hold the feet. If this is not possible, do the movements, as before, with the farthermost area of the legs you can reach.

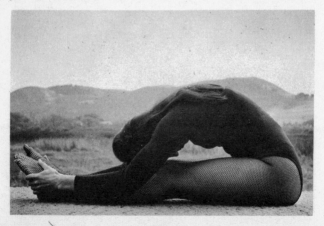

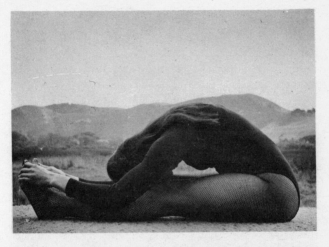

Fig. 70   The extreme position, which denotes complete flexibility of the spine. When you are eventually able to hold your feet as in Fig. 69, perform the following: After you have completed the five stretching movements of Fig. 69, do not straighten up. Instead, move your hands up to hold your toes rather than your feet. Bend your elbows as far down as you can reach for a count of five, then straighten your elbows, then lower them again. An intensive stretch in the legs and lower spine will be experienced. Do these movements five times.

Finally, straighten your trunk slowly to the upright position, rest your hands on your thighs, and relax.

Perform the entire routine of the four positions twice.

BACK STRETCH

• Most students, when they try this exercise for the first time, are unable to reach past the knees or calves. A comment I often hear is, "I can't do this exercise. I'm too stiff." Of course this is exactly why we perform these movements—to work out stiffness. A stiff, tense spine and back cannot be healthy or beautiful. The Back Stretch removes tightness, helps to firm and strengthen, and will impart a streamlined appearance to your back.

• Whereas the previous exercise, the Cobra, bends the spine *inward,* the Back Stretch moves it *outward.* A combination of the two exercises provides intensive, beneficial manipulation, especially when followed with the Plough and the Twist postures.

• Each day you will find yourself able to bend farther forward, and in a surprisingly short period of time you will be holding your ankles and then your feet. The very extreme position of Fig. 70 will take time to accomplish, but always remember that the attempt and practice are important, not how far forward you can bend.

• Whenever you perform the Back Stretch, follow all of the steps; i.e., no matter how flexible you have become, always start by holding your knees, then your calves, then working your way down your legs to your ankles and feet. These four positions manipulate the different vertebrae and work on various areas of the back. If you are unable to go farther than your knees, do the exercise several times with the knees only. If you can go as far as your calves, perform the movements several times with the knees first, then several times with your calves.

> • Remember to drop your head downward and bend your elbows outward in all of the stretching movements. Your knees should never bend.

• This exercise combines the *holds* with *continuous movements*.

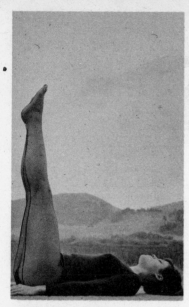

PLOUGH

Rest your back on the mat; place your arms at your sides and allow your body to go limp.

Fig. 71 Raise your legs stiffly and slowly to tone your abdominal muscles. Bring your legs to a right-angle position as illustrated.

Fig. 72 Push down hard with your palms; swing your legs back over your head and very slowly lower them as far as possible, without strain to your back, toward the floor.

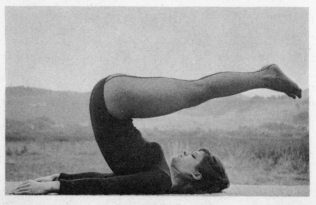

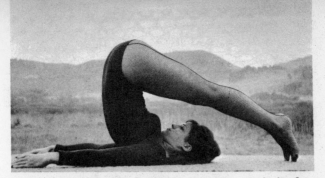

Fig. 73 The completed posture. Your feet touch the floor and your body is in the shape of a plough. Palms remain on the floor; legs are together with knees straight; chin is pressed against the chest. During the first few attempts your breathing may be irregular but this will soon adjust to normal.

When you have perfected the previous posture we can manipulate the back and spine still farther through two additional positions. You cannot continue until your feet are touching the floor with ease.

Fig. 74 Clasp your hands on the top of your head. This posture enables you to inch back slightly farther with your toes, and you will experience the emphasis shifting from your lower back (as in Fig. 73) to your middle area. Breathe slowly. Hold for a count of ten.

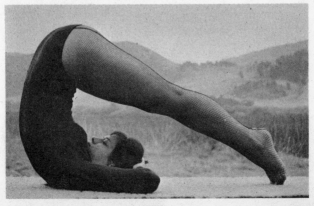

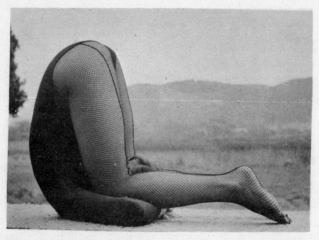

Fig. 75 Now lower your knees to either side of your head. Have them touch the floor if possible. The emphasis shifts from the middle to the upper back and neck. Hold for a count of ten. You will have to breathe very slowly.

Regardless of how far you can go with the Plough, the following are the directions for coming out of any of the positions:

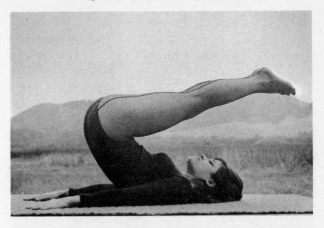

Fig. 76 Roll forward slowly, with control, until your hips touch the floor (do not tumble quickly forward). *Keep your head on the floor by arching your neck.*

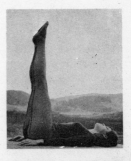

Fig. 77 Extend your legs into a right-angle position and slowly lower them to the floor. Relax completely for approximately thirty seconds.

Perform as much of the Plough routine as you can twice.

PLOUGH

• The Plough can be done directly following the Back Stretch.

• The completed posture of Fig. 73 is not easy, but it can be accomplished by simply holding whatever extreme position you attain for the count of ten. Do this twice each time you practice. The "hold" and the weight of your legs gently force the spine to "give," so that your legs can be lowered increasingly farther.

• In order to perform the movements of Figs. 74 and 75 it will be necessary to perfect the position of Fig. 73. If your feet are not touching the floor and you move your arms to clasp your hands on your head, you will tumble forward. Therefore the completed Plough must be accomplished before you can continue.

• If in Fig. 72 you have difficulty raising your hips from the floor, try swinging your legs backward rather quickly to gain the necessary momentum.

• You will realize the effectiveness of the Plough as you experience the pressure being transferred from the lower to the middle and finally to the upper back through the different positions. In this manner it is possible to manipulate thoroughly the entire back and spine.

TWIST

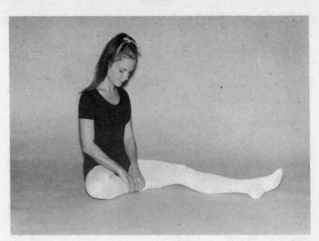

Fig. 78 Sit on the mat and extend your legs. Take your right foot with your hands and place your right heel as far in as possible.

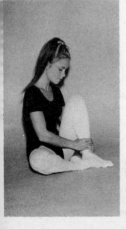

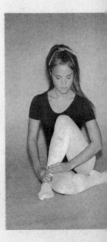

Figs. 79, 80 Hold your left ankle and swing your left leg over your right knee. The left sole rests on the floor as illustrated.

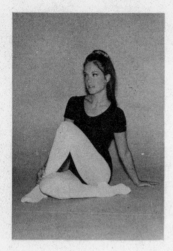

Fig. 81 Place your left hand behind you for balance.

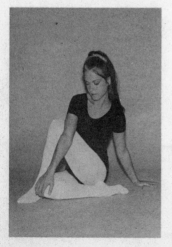

Fig. 82 Raise your right arm and bring it over your left leg so that you can hold your right knee as illustrated. Make certain your entire right arm has come over your left leg (not around it). This movement will hold the lumbar area in a straight position.

Fig. 83 Against this lock we can now twist the entire spine. Turn your head and trunk as far to the *left* as possible (make certain you turn *left*, not right); try to rest your chin on your shoulder. Reach around your waist with your left hand and attempt to hold the right side of your waist. The greater the twist and the more cramped you feel, the better. Sit with your spine erect. Hold without moving for a count of ten.

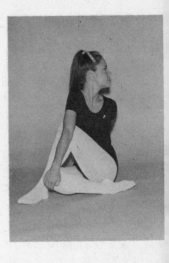

Fig. 84 A back view of the completed posture. When the count is completed, keep your arms and legs where they are but allow your trunk to turn slightly frontward. Then, without pause, twist again as far to the left as possible. In continuous motion repeat the frontward and twisting movements five times.

Turn your trunk frontward and extend your legs.

Now bring your left foot in and perform all of the identical movements on the opposite side (twisting to the *right*). Exchange the words "right" and "left" in the above directions.

Perform the Twist routine once on each side.

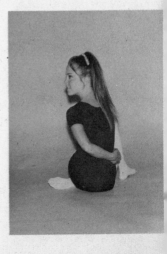

• This posture completes the Beauty for the Back series. In the previous three exercises we have methodically worked the spine inward and outward; here, the locking of the lumbar area, through an ingenious series of movements, enables us to *twist* the entire spinal column.

> • The movements are a bit intricate and require your concentration until they are mastered. It is well worth the effort.

• Do not object to being cramped or, as one student put it, "feeling like a pretzel." This is a part of the exercise. Important: If you cannot place your hand over your leg to grip your knee as instructed in Fig. 82, *push your left foot outward and away from your right knee;* then you should be able to hold your left knee as directed. The tightness and discomfort will diminish each time you practice.

> • Remember also to turn your head as far toward your shoulder as possible when twisting. This is essential to aid in the complete spinal twist.

• Students often feel highly exhilarated after this exercise, since there is an immediate loosening of the vertebrae and a great amount of energy seems to be released.

BEAUTY
FOR THE
HIPS AND THIGHS

Unnatural *Glamour*	**Natural *Beauty***
Various types of girdles and constrictive apparel to disguise shape and size; massages; appliances; calisthenics to "spot" reduce and firm.	Yoga exercises that are part of a complete program for weight control and firming.

      The bone formation of many women makes them easily prone to becoming heavy in the hips and thighs. Although it is unfortunate that a woman is ever made to feel uncomfortable concerning her natural form, the glamour industry has been so successful in fostering its concepts of "desirability" that a woman with a large bone structure has two strikes against her to start. Even if she is in her twenties and has fought a successful battle to squeeze into clothes several sizes smaller than she should naturally wear, when she reaches the age of approximately thirty she finds that she must be especially careful in her habits. This is the age at which overindulgence in food or lack of proper exercise starts to allow excess weight to settle happily in the hips, thighs, and buttocks and, once there, is determined to stay. Of course this condition can occur earlier in life or later; among my students I have found that thirty is the average age when most women, including those who until this time have had no figure problem, become aware that some real discipline will be necessary to keep the shapes they have.

The career woman, secretary, teacher, and those in other occupations that are considered "sedentary" are easily subject to the excess weight problem because of their relative inactivity. All such people should resolve to practice their Yoga routines without fail, as outlined in the Practice Plan at the end of this book. They should do this after returning home from work each day, not only to prevent excess weight and to firm up the hips and thighs, but to relieve tension and promote good blood circulation.

The housewife and mother who has been married approximately five years and has one or more young children is in a particularly vulnerable position both physically (due to the bearing of children) and psychologically. The housework routine often seems not to allow sufficient time or inclination for exercising. Also, the housewife generally feels that she gets all the exercise she needs in her housework chores and duties as a mother. This is not the case. Most of the activities in which she is involved require movements that actually *promote* stress, strain, and tension. These movements cannot be considered as methodical exercise that manipulates all parts of the body, relieves tension, and stimulates organs and glands. Despite her household activities the housewife will usually find herself gaining weight and "spreading." Therefore it is essential that she provide the time to exercise correctly. The Yoga routines, being much more enjoyable and effective than calisthenics, offer the most practical solution to the exercise problem.

Under Beauty for the Abdomen we have mentioned the temporary and deceptive help to be gained from massages and the various appliances (including, incidentally, the steam or sauna baths). We have also commented on the uncomfortable and unhealthy effects of tight girdles and other constrictive garments that attempt to disguise. These statements apply here as well. The less you must resort to the use of these artificial devices the better. Previous suggestions regarding the careful attention to be given to diet also hold true in this area. Overindulgence in food for any length of time during this period of a woman's life causes an excess-weight condition that usually proves disastrous for the hips, thighs, and buttocks. A lifetime weight battle ensues.

Therefore, if you are not experiencing a figure problem at the present time, you should undertake the Yoga practice as a *preventive* program. If you *are* in the process of "spreading," the Yoga routines can offer the most practical, sensible help for regaining your natural figure and your beauty.

The four exercises that follow are primarily for reducing and firming in the hips, thighs, and buttocks.

SIDE BEND

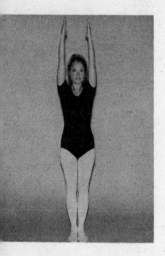

Fig. 85 Stand with your heels together and gracefully raise your arms to the position illustrated.

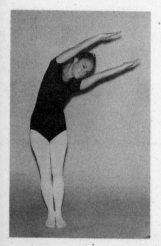

Fig. 86 Very slowly bend a moderate distance to your *left* and hold this position without motion for a count of five. It is essential that your arms remain parallel (palms facing each other) and your legs are straight. Feel a pull on your right side. When the count is completed, very slowly straighten to the upright position of Fig. 85. (The slow movement helps to tighten and firm.)

Fig. 87 Very slowly bend a moderate distance to your *right*. Hold for a count of five without moving, and make certain that your arms remain parallel. Very slowly straighten to the upright position. Bend your elbows and lower your arms several inches to relax them for a few moments. Then straighten your arms to the overhead position once again.

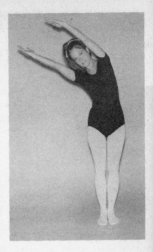

Fig. 88 Now very slowly bend as far to the *left* as you can. Keep your arms parallel; let your neck go limp; feel an intense pulling throughout the right side and into your thighs. Hold for a count of five without motion, and then perform the following movements: raise your trunk just an inch and then once again bend as far down as possible; raise the trunk slightly and bend again, etc. Do this five times, attempting to bend a fraction of an inch farther down each time. Your arms must remain parallel and your legs straight. *Make sure you are bending to the side only—do not move the trunk forward or backward.*

Straighten to the upright position, bend the elbows, and relax your arms a moment.

Now perform the extreme bend to your *right* side, all movements being identical with those of the left. Remember that first you hold your extreme position for a count of five, then perform the slight up-and-down movements five times.

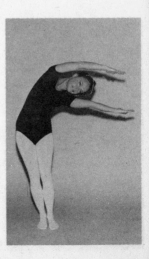

Slowly straighten to the upright position and gracefully lower your arms.

Perform the entire routine of the Side Bend twice.

95

LEG RAISE

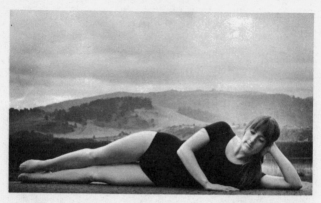

Fig. 89 Lie with your left side on the mat. Rest your head on your left palm and place your right palm firmly against the floor. Your legs are together as illustrated.

Fig. 90 Slowly raise your right leg as high as you can. Hold for a count of five. Slowly lower.

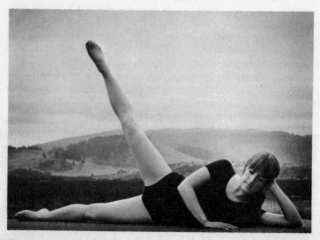

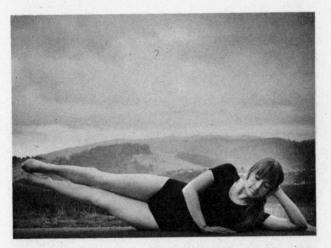

Fig. 91 Both legs are raised as high as possible. Your palm pushes down hard against the floor. *Bring your legs straight up from the side;* make sure they are kept together; do not allow them to move frontward or backward while holding for a count of five. Slowly lower and repeat. Do the identical movements on your right side, raising first your left leg once, then both legs.

Perform the Leg Raise on both sides, first raising each leg once, then both legs three times.

BACK PUSH-UP

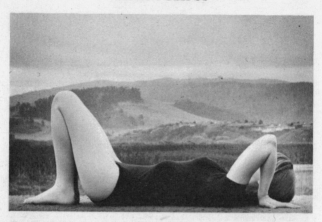

Fig. 92 Lie on your back on the mat. Carefully place your hands and your heels in the position illustrated. Your knees are together.

Fig. 93 Raise your buttocks and lower back by pushing against the floor with your hands and feet. Keep your knees and heels together. Hold for a count of ten and slowly lower to the position of Fig. 92.

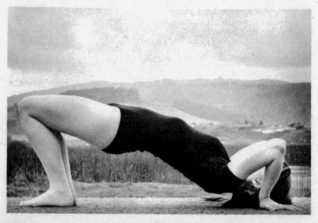

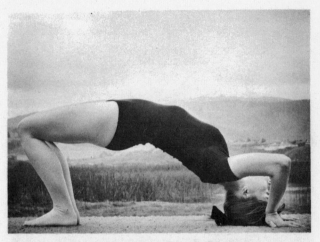

Fig. 94   Now begin to lift your entire trunk. As you do so, arch your neck and rest the top of your head on the floor. Push down hard with your hands and raise as high as possible. Keep your knees and heels together. Hold for a count of ten. Next, slowly lower your body several inches (do not come too far down) and then push up to the extreme position once again. Do these up-and-down movements five times without pause. Slowly lower to the position of Fig. 92.

Perform the Back Push-up once as in Fig. 93 to warm up and three times with the hold and up-down movements as in Fig. 94.

LEG OVER

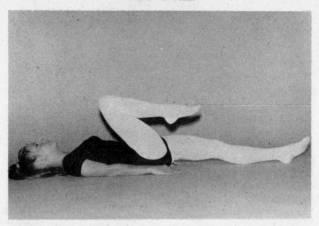

Fig. 95 Lie on your back on the mat, palms down, legs together. Bend your right knee and slowly bring it as far toward your head as possible.

Fig. 96 Gracefully raise your leg to an upright position.

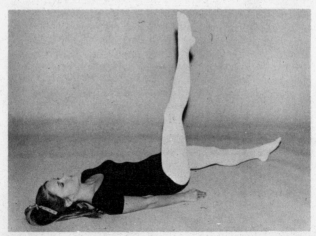

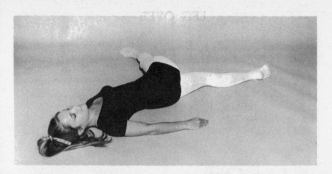

Fig. 97 (Above) Keeping both shoulders and palms on the floor, move your right leg over the left and touch your foot to the floor. Place your leg at a right angle to the trunk. Hold for a count of ten.

Fig. 98 (Below) When the count is completed, attempt to slide your right leg an inch or two farther toward your head —actually as far toward the head as it can go. Without pause, return your leg to the right-angle position. Repeat these continuous, slow-motion, up-and-down leg movements so that you do ten in all. Then return your right leg to the upright position of Fig. 96 and lower it slowly to the floor.

Do the identical movements with your left leg.

Perform the entire routine of the Leg Over exercise twice, alternating the sides, i.e., left-right, left-right.

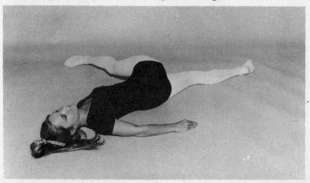

BEAUTY
FOR THE WAISTLINE

Unnatural *Glamour*	Natural *Beauty*
Calisthenics; appliances; massages; sauna and steam baths; crash diets; constrictive apparel to disguise size and shape.	An intensive series of Yoga waistline exercises to take off inches; application of the Yoga natural nutrition plan for permanent weight regulation.

The "waist" is a relatively small area located between the thorax and hips and is not to be confused with the "stomach" or "abdomen." It is possible to have developed a protruding abdomen and still be small in the waist (although probably not for long). The natural shape of the body is to be narrower in the waistline than directly above or below, and it is when this narrowness begins to disappear that a woman can be sure she is on her way to "spreading." The glamour industry has successfully promoted the idea of an exaggerated narrowness in the waistline, regardless of whether or not it is contrary to the natural bone structure of a particular woman. This campaign has led to the extraordinary sales of those undergarments that attempt to constrict, as well as dresses, suits, coats, etc., that disguise. We have already written about these things. From our Yogic viewpoint it is certainly desirable that the waist maintain its *natural* narrowness, and in this connection we must now discuss the over-all program of natural and permanent weight control.

The Weight Problem

There are very few women who do not realize the unpleasant consequences of being overweight. Most are aware of this from the standpoint of appearance, although more and more women are beginning to recognize the fact that excess weight also places their health in jeopardy. So there is no doubt as to the importance of maintaining correct weight; the question that continues to plague millions of Americans is, "How?"

The majority of people watching their weight feel they are involved in a battle. Indeed, this is exactly the case. One part of their being acts as a watchdog and must be constantly on guard against another part that is always ready to break training. Some women are able to maintain this situation through a strong self-discipline or by receiving disciplinary help from a physician, weight club, etc. Others do not fare as well; they are able to conform to their program part of the time but slip away fairly often. Still others switch from one diet and exercise plan to another, seldom able to maintain the necessary discipline.

The Dynamics of Dieting

Having been in close contact with many thousands of women who undertake these various weight-control programs, I became aware of a fascinating dynamic that seems to be almost universally present. Regardless of the temporary success of a particular program (and it is important to note that many of these are without merit, some actually being harmful), the battle that is being waged causes a continual uneasiness in which the body and mind are seldom at peace. This is due to the split that takes place between the "good" part, acting as the watchdog, and the "bad" part, being held in check. If, for example, you crave certain foods and your calorie chart says "No," you feel deprived, you wage the battle between what your body wants and what your mind says you are allowed. If your schedule calls for fifty laps on the exercise bicycle or twenty-five sit-ups and your body is simply not in the mood to do them, you must then exert a great amount of discipline to perform the necessary movements; again you wage the battle and, each time you lose, your guilt grows. The uneasiness caused by this split seems to build gradually into a real anxiety that is sometimes subtle, sometimes overt, but nonetheless culminates in a drastic modification or a complete abandonment of the program. There are many shades and degrees of the way in which this anxiety manifests itself, but the point is that of the millions of women who each year undertake an infinite number of weight-control plans, only a very, very small percentage is able to stay with and benefit from them.

To be truly effective, any program that is undertaken must be comfortable and enjoyable or, to reduce the idea to its basics, *it must feel natural*. Denial, guilt, and discipline should be absent or at a bare minimum. Almost without exception the weight-control plans that are now offered are contrary to nature. Not only the substance of these plans but the very words "weight control" are poorly chosen and provide a clue to the physical as well as the psychological difficulty. "Control" implies the identical battle discussed above. The more you attempt to "control" your weight, the more impossible it becomes to do so. You cannot, in the long run, split yourself into two parts and wage a battle. You must, on the contrary, make very good friends with yourself so that there is no split; there must be no inner watchdog. Nor should you realistically hope to depend on an external watchdog for the rest of your life.

Yoga as a Way of Life

What then shall we do? Is it possible to devise an effective diet and exercise plan in which the participant does not feel deprived, inadequate, or guilty? Our answer is, "Absolutely, but only if this program is natural, one that is not contrary to nature." This is exactly what is offered through Yoga. The practice of Yoga can become a natural way of life rather than a "program." The Yogic postures are, for the most part, natural movements that the body delights in making, as opposed to the tedious and devitalizing calisthenic-type "exercises" to which most women sooner or later become extremely resistant and which the body seldom enjoys. Indeed, Yoga has such a profound effect on the entire organism that if you should ever discontinue your Yoga practice for even a few days you will feel a definite need to resume the various stretching, relaxing, and energizing techniques—not out of guilt, but because the body itself, in its great wisdom, will want to engage in the Yoga movements. Therefore you need not force yourself to exercise. The organism, of its own accord, will bring this about. During the first few months you may have to call upon your discipline to follow the Practice Plan as outlined at the end of this book. After this initial period you will begin to look forward to your Yoga practice as one of the most enjoyable times of the day. Thereafter, for your entire life, you will seldom be able to allow more than a few days to elapse without devoting sufficient time to Yoga. *It will become a natural part of your activities.*

A Nutrition Plan for You

It is in the same natural manner that we must consider a plan of nutrition. The word "diet," like the word "control," has negative connotations. Again it implies restriction and denial. A positive approach would be to think in terms of "selecting" the foods the body really wants rather than "denying" ourselves what our eyes and taste buds desire.

We have a great, innate wisdom. In the study of Yoga we attempt to learn the art of tuning in to this wisdom. If an individual can listen with the inner ear and become truly sensitive to what her organism is saying, she will begin to live in harmony with herself; she will rely less and less on external advice—what people tell her to do —and more and more on her own profound wisdom. Just as this wisdom carries on all of the functions necessary to sustain our lives (we do not, for example, consult anyone on how to make our blood circulate), so does it know better than all the contrivers of diet plans what foods are most desirable for each of us! If a woman can become sensitive to her nutritional needs, she will find that in the same manner as her body wants to engage naturally in the Yoga movements, so will it want to abstain naturally from foods that are harmful or promote excess weight. Consequently, as with the exercises, she will not have to wage a battle to do what is necessary; the organism itself will also bring this about. She will need to consult the calorie charts and diet plans less and less and be able to trust the wisdom of her body more and more. What better approach can there be to a natural, permanent regulation of one's weight?

The Body's Nutritional Needs

Our attempt to become sensitive to the body's nutritional needs takes the form of noting its reactions to the various foods we eat. When this is done carefully, in the spirit of a scientific investigation, we begin to learn which foods make us feel heavy, listless, less alert, depressed, irritable, nervous, unable to sleep, and those that may have the opposite effects, i.e., impart vitality and promote a sense of life and well-being. You may be quite surprised to discover that many of these feelings can indeed be attributed to what we eat; that meat can drain your vitality, that coffee can depress you, that highly seasoned and spiced foods can cause insomnia, that sugar (and sugar substitutes) can make you irritable, and that all of these can have an adverse effect on your health.

Natural Foods

As you undertake this experiment of observing your body's reactions to your usual foods, we suggest that you simultaneously include in your diet a group of *natural foods*. These will be defined as those foods that are consumed as closely as possible to the way in which nature has intended. From our Yogic viewpoint foods have *life-force* (Sanskrit: *prāna*). The entire object of eating is to absorb this life-force. To the extent that foods are denatured, that is, refined, canned, preserved, frozen, smoked, aged, colored, fumigated, enriched, processed, and otherwise tampered with and prepared in a manner that renders them lifeless, they lose their value. Therefore when the Yogi selects his food the paramount consideration is: How much life-force is in this food? How *natural* is it? It has been my experience that the more a student is able to contact the wisdom of her body, the more she senses that her real nutritional requirements for both health and beauty are made up primarily of natural foods. The closer she can adhere to a natural eating plan, the better she is going to feel in both body and mind and the easier it is going to be to maintain a normal, sensible weight. Actually it is difficult to put on excess weight when you are eating naturally, because your organism will not allow you to overeat. This must be experienced to be understood.

Acceptable and Unacceptable Foods

In Yoga nutrition, as in various other diets, there are foods that are classified as acceptable and those that are considered undesirable. The principle that governs the classifications is, however, not the same. The various diet plans (and there seem to be thousands of them) are based for the most part on the consideration of substances and quantities without regard to the *quality* of these substances. For example, a diet plan may allow you x number of calories to be made up of so much fat, so much protein, so much sugar, etc. There is seldom any differentiation made between the *types* of proteins, the *types* of sugars, etc. In Yoga these distinctions are essential. There is an important difference between the quality of the protein in meat and that in nuts, cheese, mushrooms, or avocados; from our Yogic viewpoint refined table sugar or that used in candy, cake, or soft drinks is not the same as that derived from fruits, dates, or beets. Again the principle that is of primary importance to us is not how many calories there are in a particular food but rather: How *natural* are the foods that we have chosen?

Here is our standard list of natural foods that I offer to all of you.

NATURAL FOODS

DAIRY FOODS
(these are also
fats and proteins)

Milk: certified raw, non-fat, goat, evaporated

Cheese: cottage (uncreamed), farmer, ricotta, Wisconsin Cheddar

Yogurt (and all sour-milk products)

Butter (made from whole milk)

Eliminate or consume sparingly:

Homogenized, pasteurized milk
All salted, spiced, and aged cheeses
Buttermilk
Sour cream
Cream cheese
All yogurts that are flavored with fruits and syrups
Butter containing salt and animal fats

BEVERAGES

All fresh fruit and vegetable juices

Vegetable broths

Herb teas

Cereal beverages (as coffee substitutes)

Eliminate or consume sparingly:

Coffee
Tea
Alcoholic beverages
Colas and all syrup drinks
Ice cream beverages
Bottled, frozen, and canned juices

CONDIMENTS
(spices, seasonings)

All edible herbs

Vegetable salt

Eliminate or consume sparingly:

Salt and all salted products
Vinegar
All hot spices such as chili peppers

GRAINS

All whole-grain products for bread, cereal, spaghetti, crackers, etc.

Eliminate or consume sparingly:

All refined flour products such as white bread, dry cereals, most cakes and cookies, spaghetti (read the labels on these products to determine the type of flour used)

MINERALS

Apples, apricots, artichokes, beets, blueberries, broccoli, Brussels sprouts, cabbage, carrots, cauliflower, celery, cherries, cranberries, cucumbers, dandelion, eggplant, endive, garlic, grapefruit, grapes, green peas, green peppers, kale, leeks, lemons, lettuce, limes, melons, mustard greens, oranges, parsley, parsnips, peaches, pears, pineapples, plums, pomegranates, prunes, radishes, raspberries, rhubarb, spinach, squash, strawberries, string beans, tangerines, tomatoes, turnips, watercress

Eliminate or consume sparingly:

The only restrictions for fruits and vegetables are individual preference with regard to ease of digestion. Eliminate whatever is not agreeable.

OILS
(used for cooking and dressings; these are also classified as "fats")

Safflower oil

Sesame seed oil

Olive oil (pure)

PROTEINS
Avocados

Legumes (beans, peas, lentils, soy beans, and soy bean products)

Nuts (unroasted and unsalted): almonds, cashews, pecans, walnuts, Brazil nuts

Coconuts (and coconut milk)

Nut butter (almond, cashew)

Meat (organ meats preferred, particularly beef liver, kidneys, brains)

See also Dairy Foods

Eliminate or consume sparingly:

Peanuts
Meat (other than organ meats)
Poultry
Fish (those fish that feed on sea vegetables are preferable to those that eat other fish)
Crustacia (lobster, crab, shrimp)
All wafers, powders, and tablets referred to as "high-protein" products

STARCHES	SUGARS
Bananas	Fresh fruits
Brown rice	Molasses
Potatoes (baked, boiled)	Honey (uncooked, unbleached)
Whole-grain breads, crackers	Raw sugar
Pumpkin	Beet sugar
Barley	Cane sugar (the cane stalks)
Rye	Carob (St. John's bread)
	Dried fruits (dates, figs, prunes, raisins, apricots, peaches, etc., al! unsulphured)
Eliminate or consume sparingly:	*Eliminate or consume sparingly:*
White rice	All refined sugar products
Fried foods	All syrups
Pies or puddings (of the above)	All sugar substitutes referred to
Refined flour products	as "low calorie" products and used for coffee, tea, and colas.

Here are some important points for your careful consideration:

1. Substitute foods from the Natural Foods list for similar foods that have been denatured (as defined above) whenever possible.
2. Steaming, baking, and broiling are the best cooking methods for us. Avoid frying foods or using any substance that produces grease in cooking. Never boil or overcook your foods, especially vegetables. Heat them only until tenderized. Overcooking destroys life-force. Vegetables should always retain

some crispness and not be soggy. Save and use as a broth or stock all the juice produced from the cooking of vegetables. Bottled or canned fruit and vegetable juices are low in life-force.

3. Most fruits can and should be eaten raw, including the skins whenever possible. Vegetable skins also contain great nourishment. If your digestion will not permit raw fruits, then stew or bake them lightly. Never add refined sugar to fruits.

4. Fresh fruits and vegetables are always our first choice. Frozen products are a second choice when fresh produce is unavailable. We are uncertain as to the amount of life-force that remains in frozen food.

5. Dried fruits (unsulphured, read the label) such as prunes, apricots, and raisins provide an excellent source of sugar energy. If necessary they may be soaked for easier digestion.

6. Our students have found that, in general, gas, heartburn, and other digestive disturbances can be reduced or eliminated if many different types of foods are not mixed at a given meal. Foods cannot be combined indiscriminately, especially by an older person, without some discomfort usually resulting. If you experience indigestion after a meal, try to recall what foods have been mixed and thereafter avoid that combination. The fewer the number of different foods consumed at a given meal, the less the chances for indigestion. Highly spiced and seasoned foods are major offenders in digestive disturbances. Learning to combine foods so that they are easily digested is an essential factor in Yoga nutrition.

7. Meat, poultry, and fish should be eaten sparingly.

The Yogi feels that meat places a stress on the system and requires more of an expenditure of life-force in digestion than the meat itself produces. You are probably familiar with the heavy feeling in body and mind after a meat meal. Since our objective in Yoga is to remain light and alert, we must question the real value of meat. It is our belief that protein of a superior quality without the heaviness and stress of meat is obtained from natural foods as listed under Protein in our chart. This is not a subject that can be intellectually discussed or debated to advantage. To understand what is involved we suggest that the student experiment in reducing her intake of flesh foods to a minimum or eliminating them entirely for a period of thirty days. Natural proteins should be substituted. At the end of the thirty-day period the student should return to her usual quantities of meat consumption. A dramatic letdown and sluggishness are often experienced when the meat diet is resumed, and this is adequate proof to many people that the intake of meat should be strictly limited. Try this experiment and judge for yourself.

8. If you find it necessary to eat meats we suggest those in our list as being more easily digested and more nourishing. We do not consider poultry as being superior to red meat, especially in light of its quick-fattening processing. Fish is probably the most easily digested of the flesh foods. Steaming, baking, and broiling are the most acceptable cooking methods.

9. We strongly discourage the use of pills, powders, wafers, and all agents that act as appetite deter-

rents. These things may be able to fool the body temporarily but cannot result in a satisfactory solution to the permanent weight-regulation problem. We also believe that "high-protein" diets set the body on fire. In the long run they do not increase but rather deplete vitality. In effect these diets attempt to burn up excess weight, but it has been our experience that weight lost in this manner is quickly regained the moment the large amounts of protein (mostly meat, eggs, powders, wafers, etc.) are reduced. This cannot be considered an intelligent or natural method of weight regulation.

10. During this experimental period it is an excellent idea to undertake a juice fast for one or two days a week. That is, limit your food to fresh fruit juices on the selected days. If this presents a hardship, then juices are substituted for breakfast and/or lunch and one has dinner as usual. This type of moderate fasting will greatly accelerate the regulation of weight and increase one's sensitivity to what is being eaten. Advanced Yoga students often undertake a consecutive two- or three-day fast, drinking only fruit juices or distilled water. I highly recommend a moderate fasting program to every Yoga student.

11. Health food stores, some of which have shortcomings and peculiar products, are excellent places in which to obtain many natural foods. A number of them now offer produce (fruits, vegetables, dried fruits, nuts) that has not been fumigated with chemical sprays.

12. It must be stressed that people vary widely in their reactions to different foods and the combinations

thereof. For this reason it is misleading for news-papers and magazines to publish diet plans and invite great masses of readers to follow them faith-fully. Such plans may prove successful for some, although, as I have stated, most women find it ex-tremely difficult to stay with any diet even if it is temporarily successful, because it is contrary to the body's desires. The majority will find these plans disappointing and in some cases harmful. Hence our emphasis on each student becoming a law unto herself by beginning to introduce more natural foods into her food program and *carefully observing the reactions of what she is eating on her own particular, unique organism.*

13. I always urge students to keep their food experi-ments to themselves. Do not tell people you are "dieting." Everyone will give advice; some will discourage you, others will want to debate, still others will ridicule. You lose a great amount of life-force by talking about what you are doing, even to your best friends. Wait until you have ac-complished your objective and then you can speak if you wish.

14. As always, if you are under the care of a physi-cian, consult him before undertaking any of these suggestions.

15. When denatured foods are decreased and natural foods are substituted, the taste buds gradually lose their need for the various spices, seasonings, and sweeteners that are the chief attraction of the de-natured foods. In this manner you will find that, without waging a battle, it becomes natural to lose your desire for the very foods that cause digestive disturbances and excess pounds!

YOGA BEAUTY MENUS

Following are menus for one week. These are suitable for the entire family and make use of the ideas we have been discussing without being extreme. They should prove to be interesting and satisfying and constitute a new adventure in eating.

These menus may be used exactly as presented *but they are really meant to serve as examples of the types of foods and combinations that can be used.* The inventive cook will be able to devise an endless number of wholesome meals by using these menus as examples and by substituting items from our Natural Foods list. In following the menus presented, as well as those that you will create, the basic idea at all times is to note continually the reactions that the various foods and their combinations have upon you. In this way you can modify the menus as necessary. Those readers who have a weight problem should follow the example of these menus but they should eat less than is indicated, eliminating many of the starches and sweets and limiting themselves to two or even one meal per day with periodic fasting as previously discussed.

Remember that a number of the suggested foods, such as whole-grain breads and crackers, certified raw milk, raw butter, soya muffins, and whole-wheat spaghetti may have to be purchased in a health food store. But most of the foods can be obtained from your usual shopping sources.

YOGA BEAUTY MENUS

MONDAY

Breakfast

Freshly squeezed grapefruit juice

Cooked whole-wheat cereal with raisins and non-fat milk or certified raw milk or yogurt topping. If necessary sweeten with honey, molasses, or raw sugar

Beverage (coffee substitute or herb tea—use wherever beverage is given)

Lunch

A bowl of fruit in season, such as apples, grapes, peaches, pears, figs, etc., with cottage cheese, yogurt, and wheat-germ topping

Bran muffin with health jam

Beverage (as above)

Dinner

Broiled liver

Steamed beets with tops

Romaine or Chinese lettuce with yogurt dressing

Banana cake

Beverage

TUESDAY

Breakfast

Fresh orange and grapefruit sections

2 poached eggs on whole-grain (unrefined, unbleached flour) toast

Beverage

Lunch

Spanish rice (made with brown rice and seasoned with vegetable salts)

Green salad with lemon-honey dressing

Carrot juice or other beverage

Dinner

Fresh fruit salad

Broiled fresh fish

Steamed spinach

Yogurt sherbet

Beverage

WEDNESDAY

Breakfast

Unsweetened apple juice

Whole-grain dry cereal with fresh berries or raisins or
bananas

Beverage

Lunch

Fresh tomato stuffed with cottage cheese

Steamed vegetable

Whole-grain crackers with raw butter or soy margarine

Fresh fruit and beverage

Dinner

Soy bean loaf

Steamed green vegetable

Stuffed celery with cottage cheese

Custard pudding

Beverage

THURSDAY

Breakfast

Freshly squeezed orange juice

Steamed brown rice with raisins and non-fat milk or certified raw milk or yogurt topping. Sweeten as previously indicated.

Beverage

Lunch

Carrot or vegetable juice

Avocado and grapefruit salad with ricotta, farmer, or cottage cheese, and yogurt dressing

Bran muffin

Beverage

Dinner

Broiled chicken livers or other organ meat

Steamed carrots and peas

Green salad with Cheddar cheese dressing

Honey ice cream; carob cookies

Beverage

FRIDAY

Breakfast

Half grapefruit

2 boiled eggs

1 slice whole-grain toast with raw butter or soy margarine

Beverage

Lunch

Tomato juice

Salad consisting of apple, celery, raisins, green pepper, and cottage cheese, with lemon-honey dressing

Stewed fruit (dried apricots, prunes, figs) soaked in water overnight. Top with wheat germ and yogurt.

Beverage

Dinner

Cup of fresh vegetable soup

Steamed fish and Chinese vegetables

Baked cauliflower with cheese sauce

Fresh fruit compote with small serving of cashew-nut butter

Beverage

SATURDAY

Breakfast

Unsweetened grape juice

Cream of rye cereal with fresh fruit in season

Beverage

Lunch

Mushroom omelet

Rye toast

Cup of fresh fruit

Beverage

Dinner

Melon

Whole-wheat spaghetti with steamed tomato sauce

Steamed string beans

Homemade cole slaw

Date-nut bread with cream cheese

Beverage

SUNDAY

Breakfast

Dried prunes and figs (soaked overnight) with yogurt and honey

Scrambled eggs

Whole-grain toast with health jam

Beverage

Lunch

Coconut-pineapple juice

Lentil curry

Whole-grain crackers

Baked apple with honey

Beverage

Dinner

Cup of pea or lentil soup

Broiled chicken   Soya muffins

Steamed broccoli   Fruit Jell-O

Cucumber salad with yogurt dressing   Beverage

At this point you will see that all figure problems are treated in both a local and an over-all manner. That is, we emphasize specific exercises for a particular area, carefully consider eating habits, and also perform various routines of exercises that work on the entire body.

The five postures that follow are to be emphasized for waistline problems.

CIRCULAR MOTION

Read these directions completely before performing the movements. In this exercise there are three positions for bending your trunk forward and then moving it in a circular manner. These positions are: moderate, intermediate, extreme.

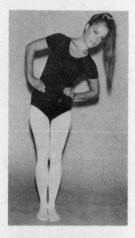

Fig. 99 In a standing posture place your hands on your hips and bend forward a few inches only so that your trunk is in the *moderate* position. We now wish to *roll and twist the trunk in a small circle* to the left, then backward, then to the right, and finally frontward. Proceed now slowly to roll and twist your trunk to the left side. Do not simply *bend* to the left—make certain that you *roll and twist* with a great amount of exaggerated motion. Hold the position for a count of five.

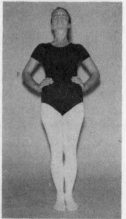

Fig. 100 In the same exaggerated motion roll and twist to the backward position. Do not go back too far; visualize your trunk as making a small circle. Hold for five.

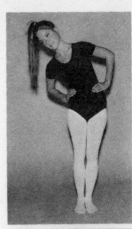

Fig. 101 In the same manner roll and twist to the right. Hold for five.

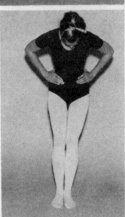

Fig. 102 Slowly roll and twist to the frontward position, keeping the small circle in mind. Hold for five.

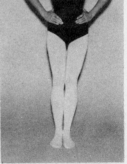

Fig. 103 Bend forward a few more inches into the *intermediate* position. Now make a wider (intermediate) circle in rolling and twisting the trunk.

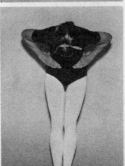

125

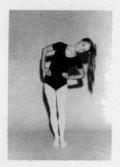

Fig. 104 Slowly roll and twist to the left in a wider circle. Do not simply bend; *roll and twist.* Hold for five.

In the same exaggerated motion roll and twist to the intermediate backward position and then to the right and frontward positions. Hold each for a count of five.

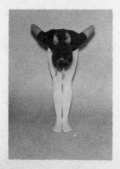

Fig. 105 Bend forward as far as you can to the *extreme* position.

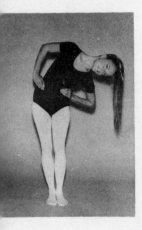

Fig. 106 Making the widest circle possible, roll and twist to the left. Hold for a count of five. When the count is completed, attempt to bend a fraction of an inch farther down on the left side. Then, without pause, raise your trunk slightly and repeat these down-and-up movements so that you do five in all.

Now roll and twist to the backward position and hold for five. When the count is completed, attempt to bend a fraction of an inch farther backward. Do this cautiously. Then raise your trunk slightly and bend backward again. Repeat these backward-and-forward movements so that you do five in all.

Next roll and twist to the right side and perform the identical movements as on the left, including the five down-and-up movements.

Finally, roll and twist forward and hold for five.

Straighten up slowly and rest.

Perform the entire Circular Motion routine, which includes rolling and twisting from the three different positions, twice.

TRIANGLE

Stand erect, arms at your sides and heels together.

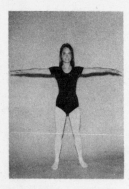

Fig. 107 Separate your legs so that they are approximately two feet apart. Raise your arms gracefully, palms facing downward.

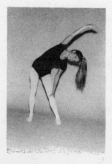

Fig. 108 Bend slowly to the left and hold your knee as illustrated. (Do not go farther than the knee.) Bring your right arm far over without bending your elbow. Feel the right side tightening. Hold for a count of five. Then straighten slowly to the upright position of Fig. 107. Your arms are again outstretched and your knees remain straight throughout the exercise.

Fig. 109 Bend to the *right* side and do the identical movements, holding your right knee for a count of five. Straighten slowly to the upright position.

Now move your legs farther apart so that the stance is considerably wider than in Fig. 107.

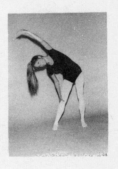

Fig. 110 Bend to the left side once again, and this time hold your calf. (Do not go farther than the calf.) Bring your right arm far over. Remember that the elbow must not bend. The pull in your right side and legs will be more intense than before. Hold for a count of five. Slowly straighten up.

Perform the identical movements on the *right* side. Hold your calf for a count of five. Slowly straighten up. Keep your legs where they are, but lower your arms to the sides gracefully and rest them for several moments. Now move your legs to form the widest stance possible. Raise your arms once again.

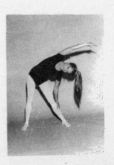

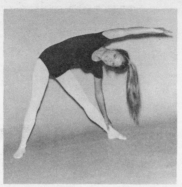

Fig. 111 This is the extreme position. Bend to the left, and this time attempt to hold your ankle without bending your knees. Bring your right arm over as far as possible, keeping the elbow straight. You will now experience an extreme pull on the side and in your legs. Hold for five without motion. Then grasp the ankle very firmly and attempt to pull your trunk down an additional inch. Bend the left elbow to help you pull down. Without pause raise your trunk very slightly, then pull down once again. Repeat these down-and-up movements so that you do five in all. Slowly straighten up.

Do the identical movements on the *right* side, first holding without motion for a count of five and then performing the down-and-up pulls. Note the triangles formed with both legs and the floor and with your arm and leg. When the five pulls are completed, straighten up slowly, lower the arms gracefully, and bring your legs together.

The entire Triangle routine, which includes holding the three areas of the leg, should be performed three times, alternating the sides.

STANDING TWIST

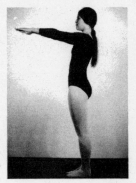

Fig. 112 In a standing posture, with your legs a few inches apart, bring your arms into the position illustrated. Palms face downward.

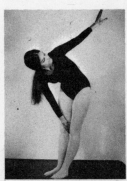

Fig. 113 Slowly bend forward. Bring your right hand down to hold the *back* of your right knee (do not go farther than the knee). Your left arm is behind you, and you turn your head and twist your trunk to look at the back of your left hand. Make sure you are holding the *back*, not the side, of your right knee. Count to five. Slowly straighten up and bring your arms back to the position of Fig. 112.

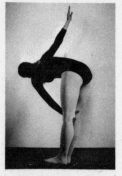

Fig. 114 Perform the identical movements on the opposite side. Your left hand holds your left knee, and you twist to see the back of your right hand. Hold for five. Slowly straighten to the position of Fig. 112.

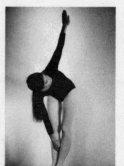

Fig. 115 Now bend forward and hold your right *calf*. Grasp it firmly so that you may now twist against the hold and once again see the back of your left hand. This time the twist will be more intense. Do not bend your knees. Hold for five. Straighten up slowly. Your arms are outstretched as you raise your trunk.

Perform the identical movements on the opposite side, holding your left calf (do not go farther than the calf) with your left hand and twisting to see the back of your right hand. Straighten up once again to the position of Fig. 112.

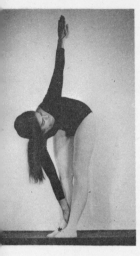

Fig. 116 The extreme position. Study the illustration. Your right hand is now firmly holding your right *heel*. Your trunk is twisted and your head is turned so that you attempt to see the back of your left hand. Do not bend your knees. When the count of five is completed, make a strong effort to twist your trunk another fraction of an inch to the left, then without pause relax your trunk and then without pause twist again. Do five of these extreme twisting movements in continuous motion. Slowly straighten to the position of Fig. 112.

Perform the identical movements holding your *left* heel and looking at the back of your right hand. Hold for five, then do the five extreme twisting movements to the right.

Straighten slowly to the position of Fig. 112. Gracefully lower your arms.

Perform the entire routine of the Standing Twist, which includes holding the three areas of the leg, twice. Alternate the sides.

STANDING TWIST

Important notes

• This is very much a dance exercise, and you should execute the movements gracefully with poise and balance.

> • If you cannot hold your heel in Fig. 116, the calf will be adequate. However, if you are unable to see your hand behind you when you twist, you are bending too far down. You must always be able to see your hand.

• Make certain that your hand holds the *back* of your knee and calf and then your heel. Some students erroneously hold the side of their leg.

> • Carefully note the words "right" and "left" as applied to the legs in the directions. Otherwise you may hold the wrong leg when performing the twisting movements. Also be sure that your knees do not bend at any point during this exercise.

• These twisting movements are unsurpassed for streamlining the waist.

ELBOW-TO-KNEE

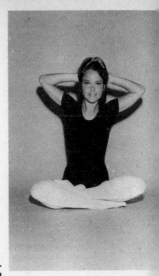

Fig. 117 Sit in a cross-legged posture and clasp your hands behind your head.

Fig. 118 Bend to your left very slowly and attempt to touch your left elbow to your left knee. If this is too difficult, go as far as possible. Hold for five. Keep both knees on the floor. When the count is completed, attempt to bend an inch farther down to the left; without pause raise your trunk slightly. Do five of these down-and-up stretches. Return slowly to the up-right position of Fig. 117.

Perform the identical movements on the right side. Straighten up.

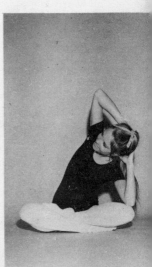

135

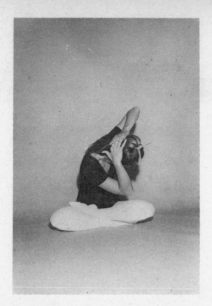

Fig. 119 In the upright position twist your trunk as far to the left as possible. Bend down very slowly and attempt to touch your left knee or calf with your *right* elbow. Study the illustration. Both knees are on the floor and the left elbow is pointing upward (this gives you the maximum stretch). Hold for five. When the count is completed, attempt to twist a fraction of an inch farther to the left; without pause relax your trunk, then twist again. Do five of these extreme twisting movements. Slowly straighten to the position of Fig. 117. Perform the identical movements on the left side. Slowly straighten up.

Perform the entire Elbow-to-Knee routine three times, alternating the sides.

SHOULDER STAND

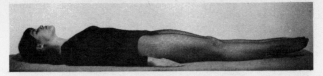

Fig. 120 (Above) Lie on your back on the mat; place your hands at your sides, palms downward.

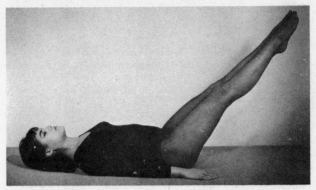

Fig. 121 (Above) Raise your legs stiffly and slowly.

Fig. 122 (Below) Push down hard with your hands and swing your legs back over your head. When your lower back leaves the floor, place your hands firmly against your hips as illustrated.

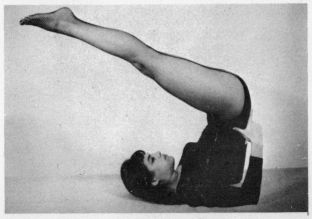

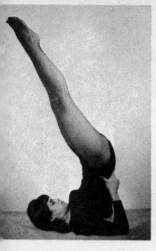

Fig. 123 Supporting your hips with your hands, straighten your trunk and legs upright as far as possible. This illustration depicts an intermediate position of the Shoulder Stand and is as far as you may be able to go in the beginning.

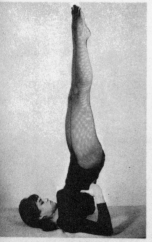

Fig. 124 The completed posture. Study the illustration. Note that your trunk and legs form a right angle with your head. In this position your chin will be pressed against your chest. Attempt to breathe slowly and rhythmically. This posture, or that of Fig. 123, is held in a *relaxed* manner from thirty seconds to five minutes, depending on your degree of accomplishment. This is the longest hold in our Yoga practice.

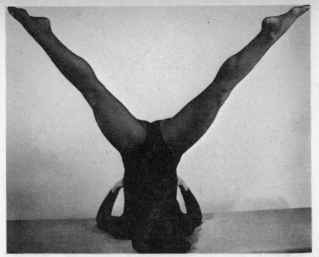

Fig. 125   When the holding time has elapsed, slowly separate your legs as far as possible. Hold this position for a count of ten.

Fig. 126   Now very slowly twist your trunk as far to the left as possible, keeping your legs apart. Your legs are actually held stationary; it is your trunk that twists. Hold the extreme twist for a count of ten.

Maintain your legs as they are and very slowly twist as far to the right as possible. Hold for ten. Twist to the frontward position of Fig. 125. Bring your legs together once again as in Fig. 124.

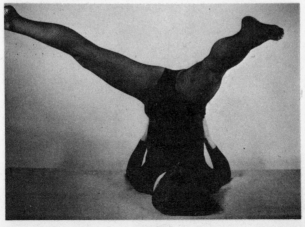

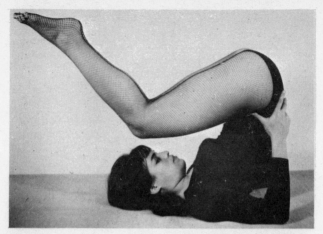

Fig. 127   Bend your knees and lower them toward your head. This movement will enable you to place your palms back on the floor.

Fig. 128   Arch your neck as illustrated and roll forward slowly, with control, until your hips touch the floor (do not tumble quickly forward). Extend your legs into the right-angle position and slowly lower them to the floor. Relax completely for approximately one minute.

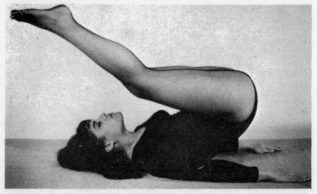

Perform the entire Shoulder Stand routine, including the left and right twisting movements, once.

SHOULDER STAND

Important notes

• The thyroid gland is an important factor in the control of weight. The major objective of the Shoulder Stand is to bring an increased flow of blood into the neck area and stimulate the thyroid gland. When this occurs, Yoga students often experience a loss of pounds and inches as well as a redistribution of weight!

• Consequently, the longer one can hold the completed (or intermediate) Shoulder Stand without strain, the greater the benefits. Begin by holding the extreme position for thirty seconds and gradually work up to three minutes and longer. It will be necessary to glance at a watch or clock placed nearby. Be exact in your timing.

• As with the Plough exercise, if in Fig. 122 you have difficulty raising your hips from the floor, swing your legs backward quickly to gain the necessary momentum.

• Straighten up into the extreme position as best you can. Whatever angle you are able to attain will be beneficial. If you are exceptionally heavy or overweight you may need to use the wall as an aid. Lie on your back, place your feet against the wall, and attempt actually to "walk up" the wall so that your hips are raised from the floor. Then hold the raised position with your feet braced against the wall for as long as is comfortable. The more overweight you are, the more essential it is to do some position of the Shoulder Stand (subject always to the approval of your physician if you are in doubt).

• A small pillow or folded towel placed beneath the neck before beginning will relieve excess pressure in the extreme position.

• Breathing must be slow and controlled; your eyes may be closed.

• The extreme positions are held in a *relaxed* fashion. There is no need to be rigid.

• Be aware also that the Shoulder Stand imparts relaxation to the legs as well as to many organs and glands. We temporarily relieve the stress of gravity in the inverted posture.

• When you have returned to the horizontal position, allow yourself to go completely limp for one minute. You will experience a deep revitalization.

BEAUTY
FOR THE LEGS

Unnatural *Glamour*	**Natural *Beauty***
Calisthenics; appliances and gadgets (such as the pedaling devices); cosmetics; an endless offering of easily damaged hose and quickly outmoded shoes.	Yoga techniques to strengthen, firm, relieve tension, take off inches, develop balance and poise.

The majority of the Yoga exercises presented here includes various movements for the legs. These movements will accomplish what is listed above under Natural Beauty. Certain of the stretching postures can actually lengthen the legs and improve their shape. There is no better system of movements, including swimming and ballet, for developing the over-all beauty of the thighs, calves, and feet.

Calisthenics for the legs, as well as the various gadgets that are used (bicycle machines, etc.), are concerned almost exclusively with an attempt to reduce inches and to firm. There is seldom any consideration given to other important factors that lend beauty to the legs. For example, stiffness and tension in the legs must be periodically removed. We accomplish this in Yoga through

143

slow-motion stretching. The value of the stretching movements will be readily appreciated by all those sedentary workers who spend most of the day sitting at their desks or who do a great deal of continual short walking. These short walks promote stress and are extremely tiring. Most housewives also have this problem. A few minutes spent after work with the Yoga exercises that follow can revitalize your legs and give them back their "spring." Various leg pains and cramps have been remarkably relieved through these stretching postures.

Exercises such as the Shoulder Stand (given under Beauty for the Waistline) and the Plough (under Back), as well as the Head Stand postures, place the legs in a position where the blood is reversed. This has proven to be most relaxing as well as helpful in artery, vein, and blood vessel problems that mar the beauty of the legs.

Develop Grace and Agility

The exercises in this section, as well as those under Balance and Poise, help the legs to develop the grace and agility that enhance their beauty in walking and other movements. It is extremely interesting to note also that certain of the leg exercises, such as the Alternate Leg Stretch, aid in balancing the sides (one leg is often slightly shorter than the other). This lends a more symmetrical feeling and appearance to the entire body.

The knees, ankles, and feet require methodical exercise for both their health and their appearance. It is important to remove stiffness and maintain strength and flexibility in these areas. The Knee and Thigh Stretch, Backward Bend, Lotus postures, and those exercises under Balance and Poise will provide the needed movements. Always remember that no part of the organism can feel or appear beautiful if there is pain, stiffness, tightness, cramp, or general discomfort. The knees, ankles, and feet are particularly subject to these, and that is why we must include the following exercises for them.

The shoes worn by many women during the greater part of the day are, of course, deadly for the feet. They deform, squeeze, cause growths, shorten the muscles, weaken the ankles, and are completely uncomfortable. Nonetheless the glamour industry has succeeded in making them standard equipment and the woman, as usual, is the loser. You should wear this standard equipment only when absolutely required. Otherwise give your feet as much freedom as possible; remove your shoes whenever you can.

An organic cosmetic can be used to maintain the smoothness of the legs.

LEG CLASP

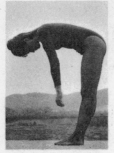

The objective of this exercise is to strengthen and firm your legs in their various areas through three stretching patterns.

Fig. 129 **Stand erect with your heels together. Slowly bend forward and bring your arms down as illustrated.**

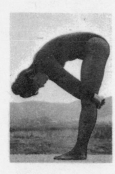

Fig. 130 **Clasp your hands firmly behind your knees (do not go farther down than the knees).**

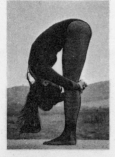

Fig. 131 **Brace your hands against the backs of your knees and slowly draw your trunk down so that your head comes as far down toward your knees as possible. Hold motionless for a count of ten. Relax your trunk but retain the clasp.**

Fig. 132 Slide your clasped hands down so that they are now braced against the backs of your calves (do not go farther than the calves). Gently draw down once again, this time aiming your head lower, more toward your calves if possible. Hold for a count of ten. Relax your trunk but retain the clasp.

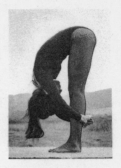

Fig. 133 The extreme posture. Your clasped hands are now as low as you can bring them—to your heels if possible. Gently draw your trunk and head down as illustrated. Hold for ten. Naturally if this is too difficult simply hold whatever extreme position you can attain. When the count is completed raise your trunk slightly and then without pause draw down again as far as possible. Repeat these down-and-up movements so that you do five in all. Unclasp your hands and very slowly straighten to the erect position.

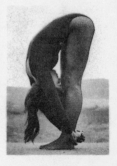

Perform the entire routine of the Leg Clasp, moving to the three leg positions, twice.

DANCER'S POSTURE

This is an intensive firming movement for the legs. It must be done with all the balance and poise of a ballet dancer.

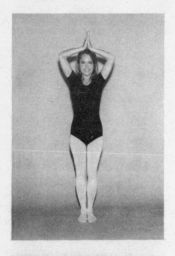

Fig. 134 You may have seen oriental dancers assume this posture. Your palms are firmly together.

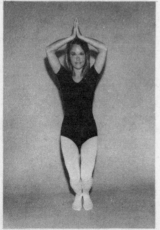

Fig. 135 Bend your knees and *very slowly* begin to lower. It is essential to keep your knees together for maximum benefits.

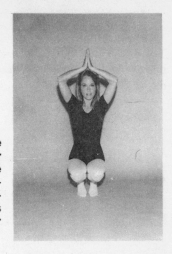

Fig. 136 As you continue to lower your trunk, your heels will automatically be raised, with your toes remaining on the floor. Attempt to have your buttocks touch your heels. Keep your knees together.

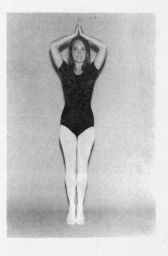

Fig. 137 Without pause raise your body as slowly as you lowered and, remaining on your toes (do not allow your heels to touch the floor again), come into the position illustrated. You will be as high on your toes as possible. Without pause lower your heels to the floor so that you are in the beginning position of Fig. 134. Without pause begin to lower once again and repeat the movements.

Perform the Dancer's Posture five to ten times. There are no "holds" in this exercise; it is done in continuous motion.

DANCER'S POSTURE

• It is important to become a dancer in this exercise and attempt to experience the beauty and symmetry of the body in motion.

> • If you lose your balance at any point, stop your movements. Immediately assume the starting position of Fig. 134 and begin again. Do not laugh or allow yourself to feel inadequate. Simply begin again. You will quickly gain the necessary skill to lower and raise slowly and smoothly.

KNEE AND THIGH STRETCH

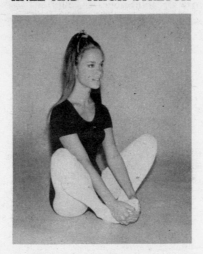

Fig. 138 In a seated posture, with your spine absolutely straight, clasp your feet and draw them in as far as possible. The soles are together.

Fig. 139 Brace your hands firmly against your feet so that your knees can be lowered.

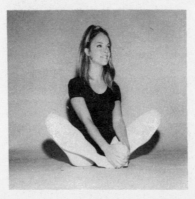

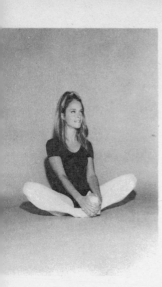

Fig. 140 The extreme position. Here your knees rest as close to the floor as possible. Your spine is held erect. If this position is difficult, hold whatever extreme posture you can attain for a count of ten.

When the count is completed allow your knees to be raised slightly from their extreme position and then without pause lower them again as far as possible. Do five of these continuous up-and-down movements. Unclasp your hands and extend your legs straight out.

The Knee and Thigh Stretch is usually performed only once. However, in cases of extreme stiffness of the knees or flabbiness of the thighs, perform the above movements, including the five continuous stretches, three times.

KNEE AND THIGH STRETCH

Important notes

• This outward stretching of your knees provides excellent relief of tension for the entire knee-thigh area. It helps make the knees limber and the thighs firm.

• Make certain your heels are drawn in as far as possible, and never allow your trunk to slump.

• You may not be able to lower your knees as far as depicted in Fig. 140, or possibly not as far as in Fig. 139. This can be due to an excessive tightness in the thighs that will gradually diminish. Do not be discouraged, and practice faithfully. Remember that limberness imparts a natural beauty to the legs.

ALTERNATE LEG STRETCH

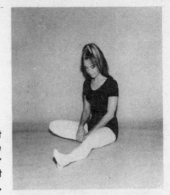

Fig. 141 Sit on the mat and extend your legs. Take your right foot with your hands and place your right heel as far in as possible.

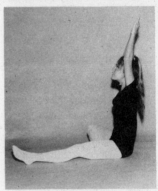

Fig. 142 In a slow, graceful movement raise your arms and bring them overhead as illustrated. Bend backward a short distance.

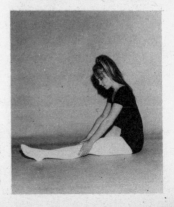

Fig. 143 Execute a slow-motion dive forward and take a firm hold on your left knee with both hands. Do not go farther than the knee.

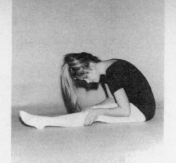

Fig. 144 Pull against your knee, bend your elbows outward, and gently draw your trunk down, aiming your forehead toward your left knee. Pull down as far as you can without strain and hold *without moving* for a count of five. Do not bend your left knee.

When the five count is completed, continue to hold your knee firmly but straighten your trunk an inch or two. Now once again pull your trunk down toward your knee, and when you have gone as far down as possible, without pause straighten your trunk an inch or two. Without pause pull down again. Repeat these short up-and-down movements so that you do five in all.

Fig. 145 Slowly straighten up and, as you do so, bring your arms overhead once again. Slowly begin to dive forward as before, this time gently rocking or swaying to and fro as you come down.

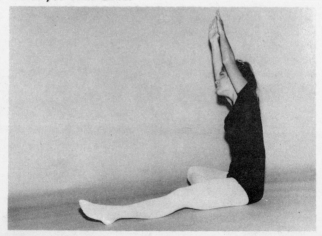

Fig. 146 Now attempt to take a firm hold on your left calf. Do not go farther than the calf. Pull against your calf, bend your elbows outward, and gently draw your trunk down, again aiming your forehead toward your left knee or calf. Do not bend your knee. Hold your extreme position for a count of five.

Continue to hold your calf firmly but raise your trunk an inch or two. Without pause pull down again and perform the up-and-down movements five times slowly, as before. If you are unable to reach your calf, simply hold your knee as in Fig. 144 and repeat the identical movements.

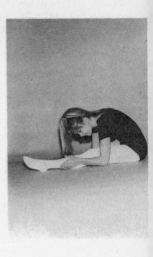

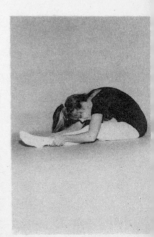

Fig. 147 Slowly straighten to the upright position, raise your arms overhead, perform the rocking movements again, and this time attempt to hold your left ankle. Draw down, hold for five, perform the short up-and-down stretches five times. If you cannot reach your ankle, simply hold your knee or calf and repeat the identical movements.

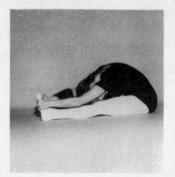

Fig. 148 Slowly straighten up and once again perform the rocking movements, this time reaching very far forward and attempting to hold your left foot with both hands. If this is not possible, do the movements, as before, with the farthermost area of your leg you can reach. Include the five short up-and-down stretches.

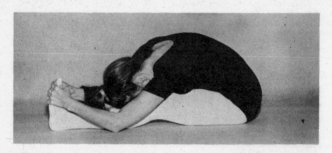

Fig. 149 This is the extreme position, which has an intense effect on the leg. With practice you will eventually be able to hold your foot as in Fig. 147 and then the following movements are performed: After you have completed the five stretching movements of Fig. 69, do not straighten up. Instead, bend your elbows as far down as you can reach for a count of five, then straighten your elbows, then lower them again. Do this five times. This movement places an intense pressure on your calf.

Finally, straighten your trunk very slowly to the upright position.

Extend your right leg straight out.

Now perform the identical movements with your *right* leg, exchanging the words "right" and "left" in the above directions.

Do the entire routine of the Alternate Leg Stretch, including the five extra stretching movements in each of the four positions, twice. Alternate the sides.

ALTERNATE LEG STRETCH

Important notes

• This is the finest exercise to relieve that tired and crampy feeling and put the "youthful spring" back in your legs. Try this one the next time you have been on your feet all day and need to revitalize.

> • You will notice a pronounced difference in the legs. That is, on one side the movements will be easier than the other. This indicates a certain unevenness in the body structure, which eventually may be corrected through the Alternate Leg Stretch.

• Again, as in many of the previous exercises, you go only as far as you can without strain. If it is too difficult to reach your foot, simply perform the movements with your knee, calf, and ankle; if your ankle is too difficult, work with your knee and calf only, etc. There is absolutely no necessity to get farther down on the leg immediately. This will come in time. Indeed, if you strain to accomplish a more extreme position than that for which you are ready you are actually retarding your progress. Remember this principle.

• Your elbows always bend outward in the pulls and your neck goes limp.

> • The Alternate Leg Stretch has proven to be a great blessing for thousands of housewives, office workers, and career women who have had various leg problems. You should be able to detect an increased vitality after one week of practice.

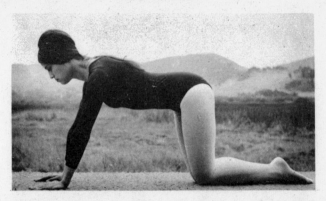

Fig. 150 Place your palms and knees on the mat. Your toes rest on the floor as depicted.

Fig. 151 Push down against the floor with your palms and toes and arch your body. Lower your head as far as possible toward the floor. Hold without motion for a count of ten.

When the count is completed, move your toes in several inches so that the arch is more acute. Your toes rest on the floor. Hold for ten.

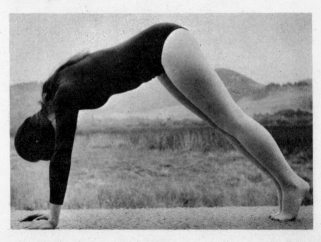

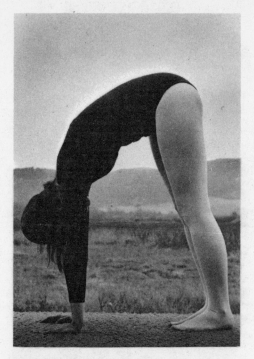

Fig. 152 The extreme position. The feet are now moved in as far as possible, and you attempt to lower the heels to touch the floor. There is an intensive stretching of your legs. Hold for ten.

Lower your knees to the floor and relax a few moments.

Move your feet back to the position of Fig. 150 and repeat the three movements.

Perform the All Fours routine twice.

LOTUS POSTURES

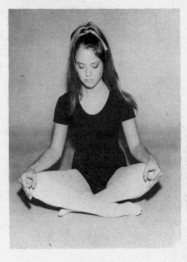

Fig. 153 The simple cross-legged posture. Your ankles are crossed and your heels drawn in as far as possible. Your wrists rest on your knees. This is a perfectly satisfactory position which beginners can assume to perform those exercises where a cross-legged posture is indicated. Do not be concerned if your knees are raised a considerable distance from the floor. They will gradually lower. Try to keep your trunk erect.

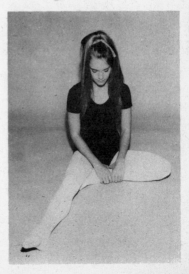

Fig. 154 Preparation for the Half-Lotus posture. First both legs are extended. Then your hands place your left heel as far in as possible.

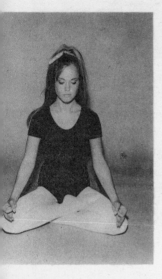

Fig. 155 The completed Half-Lotus. Your hands have now placed your right foot in the cleft of your left calf. Your right knee should rest as close to the floor as possible. Your spine is absolutely straight but your trunk remains relaxed. There is no tension in your body; this is important. Your hands assume a classical position in which the sides of your wrists rest on your knees and your index fingers press firmly against the second joint of your thumbs. When the Lotus postures are used for meditation the eyelids are lowered (but not closed). The position will be held for different periods of time as indicated in the various exercises.

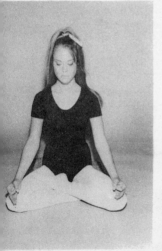

Fig. 156 The Half-Lotus with the legs reversed. Both positions should be practiced. If your knees cannot touch the floor in either position of the Half-Lotus you will not, at present, be able to execute the Full-Lotus. Therefore continue to work with the Half-Lotus until your knees are eventually lowered to the floor.

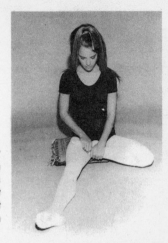

Fig. 157 Preparation for the Full-Lotus. First both legs are extended. Then your hands place your left foot on top of your right thigh with your heel drawn in as far as possible.

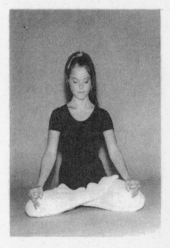

Fig. 158 The completed Full-Lotus. Your hands have placed your right foot on your left thigh with your right heel drawn in as far as possible. The spine, trunk, hand, and eye positions are identical to those of the Half-Lotus.

Attempt also to perform the Full-Lotus with the legs reversed.

There are three variations that can be attempted once the Lotus is mastered. These are more difficult postures and are presented, on the following pages, solely as a challenge to more advanced students.

163

Fig. 159 (Top) The Raised Lotus. Your hands are placed on either side and your body raised and lowered five times in continuous motion as *slowly and smoothly* as possible. This is an advanced exercise in strength and control.

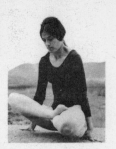

Fig. 160 (Center) This posture is named Yoga Mudra and the movements may be done in either the Half- or Full-Lotus. Sit in the erect position with hands clasped behind your back. Your trunk bends forward until the top of your head rests on the floor. Your arms are brought straight upward into the position illustrated. Note the beautiful symmetry and form of the body. This posture is actually a relaxing one once it is mastered and can be held for thirty seconds.

Fig. 161 (Bottom) The Lotus Shoulder Stand. Seated in the Full-Lotus position, lower your back to the floor and at the same time swing your legs into the position illustrated. Bring your palms up to support your hips. Hold for a count of thirty. Then lower your legs, simultaneously raising your trunk and returning to the seated position.

This posture can be considered as one of the variations of the Shoulder Stand and is performed by some students following the movements of Fig. 126. In this case your hands must be used to place your feet in the necessary position. After the hold of thirty your legs are unlocked and returned to the upright Shoulder Stand position. Then proceed to the movements of Fig. 127.

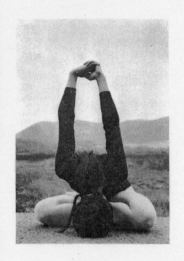

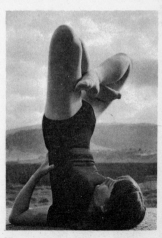

BACKWARD BEND

This exercise has three positions that provide a very thorough workout for the ankles, feet, and toes. It strengthens, imparts flexibility, and helps remove stiffness and cramps, thus counteracting, in part, the damaging effect of most shoes.

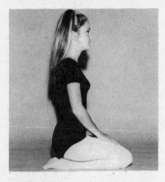

Fig. 162 Sit on your heels. Your knees are together, arms at sides.

Fig. 163 Place your palms on the floor behind you and slowly inch them backward as far as possible. Keep your knees together. Note that your hands are fairly close together and your fingers point directly behind you.

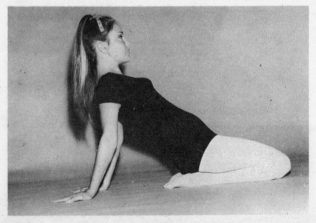

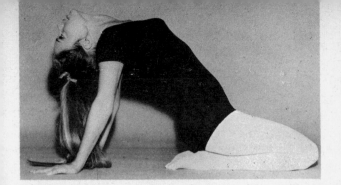

Fig. 164 Your spine is arched acutely, and your head drops as far back as possible. Do not raise your buttocks from your heels. Keep your knees together. Hold the position for a count of twenty. Move your hands in and return to the position of Fig. 162.

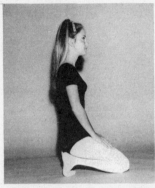

Fig. 165 Now rest your toes on the floor as illustrated.

Fig. 166 Inch back carefully as far as possible; lower your head. The curvature of the spine will now be more intense, since the trunk is higher. Remember the correct hand position. Hold for a count of twenty. If you cannot, at present, perform the next stage of the Backward Bend, return to the position of Fig. 165 and proceed to the next exercise.

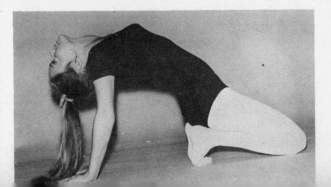

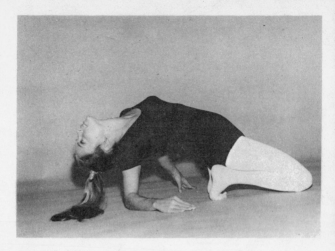

Fig. 167 Cautiously lower your right elbow to touch the floor.

Fig. 168 Lower your left elbow to the floor and hold your feet.

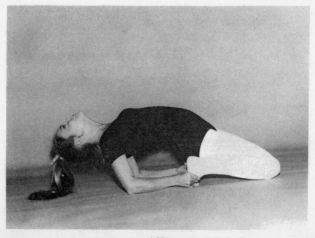

Fig. 169 The extreme posture completed. Your head is lowered to rest on the floor. Hold for ten.

To come out of this posture, release the feet, place the palms on the floor, and gently roll your body to the left so that you can extend your right leg, then your left. Raise your trunk to the upright position.

Perform as much of the Backward Bend routine as you can, once.

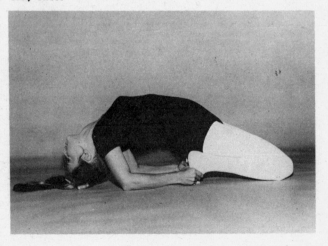

BACKWARD BEND

• The position of Fig. 164 should not be difficult unless your feet have become exceptionally stiff. In this event a little patient practice will bring good results.

• The completed position of Fig. 166 necessitates strength and flexibility of your toes. Simply sitting in the position of Fig. 165 for several seconds each day without attempting the backward movements will gradually build up the strength required. Most students must accomplish this position in stages, carefully moving their hands farther backward an additional inch each few days. You must move cautiously into the extreme position; never lunge backward.

• Fig. 169 represents an advanced Yoga posture, and many months of sustained practice are generally required before it is mastered. You should attempt this advanced position only when Fig. 166 is no longer a challenge.

Beauty for the Arms

The beauty of the arms is contingent on their correct proportion (in accordance with natural bone structure), firmness (good muscle tone), suppleness (absence of stiffness and knots in the joints and muscles), good condition of the skin (through proper nutrition and correct care), and gracefulness in movement.

The things that we wish to accomplish with regard to the shoulders, arms, wrists, and hands occur through our *over-all* Yoga practice. That is, the practice of the various exercises includes the arms to the extent that no separate grouping need be given for them. Specifically the exercises that are listed in our other sections and that emphasize the various areas of the arms most intensely are:

Back Push-Up	Bow	Hand Clasp
Backward Bend	Chest Expansion	Head Stand
Bust Exercise	Cobra	Lotus

You may devote extra time to these exercises as necessary for dealing with problems indicated above. Heaviness in the upper arms should decrease through continued practice and following the nutrition plan. Flabbiness in the upper arms, weakness, and stiffness in the elbows, wrists, and fingers respond well to these exercises. You will find that your arms automatically develop gracefulness in movement and, as is the case with your legs, often become slightly longer. Again, to maintain a smooth condition of the skin an organic cosmetic may be used as necessary.

CHAPTER 12

BEAUTY THROUGH BALANCE AND POISE

The ability to move gracefully, in a natural manner, is one of the most distinguishing characteristics of true beauty. We are not speaking here of the stilted movements of the fashion models or those of the girls who have been taught how to walk in finishing school. Such movement is artificial, extremely uncomfortable, and the very opposite of the flowing, rhythmic motion that we seek to cultivate in Yoga.

At this point you are undoubtedly aware that a number of the Yoga exercises impart a strong sense of poise. The postures make you move rhythmically, loosen your spine and joints to eliminate rigidity, improve your posture, and, as in the Alternate Leg Stretch, help to balance the sides. These accomplishments result in lifelong beauty of movement.

The three postures that follow contain many benefits, but primarily, in attempting to master the positions, you will develop a secure sense of poise and balance. Remember that beauty of movement cannot be faked; it is the expression of a body that is naturally supple and balanced.

TOE TWIST

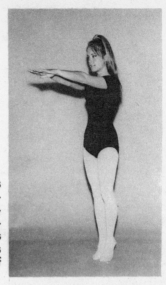

Fig. 170 Slowly raise as high on your toes as possible, simultaneously bringing your arms into the position illustrated. Your hands are touching and your eyes fixed steadily on the tips of your fingers.

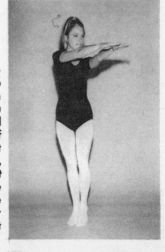

Fig. 171 Very slowly begin to twist your trunk to the left. Stay as high on your toes as possible. If you lose your balance and come down on the soles of your feet, pause a moment to gain your equilibrium, raise on your toes again at *the point where the balance was lost,* and continue the twisting movement. Your arms must always be at eye level.

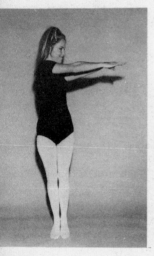

Fig. 172 The completed posture with your trunk twisted as far as possible. Note that your spine is held straight; this is important. Your eyes remain gazing at the back of your hands. Stay high on your toes although your legs may be shaky. Gradually your balance will be stabilized and you will perform these movements with the smoothness of a ballet dancer. There is no hold in this exercise. As soon as the extreme position is reached you begin to return frontward in the same slow-motion pace. When the frontward position is reached, you continue the identical movements to the *right* side.

When you have returned frontward from the right side, you lower your feet and your arms, rest for a few moments without fidgeting, and repeat the movements to the left and right sides.

Perform the entire routine of the Toe Twist three times.

BALANCE POSTURE

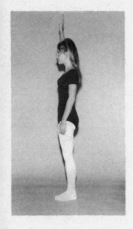

Fig. 173 (Left) Stand with your heels together and raise your right arm to the position illustrated.

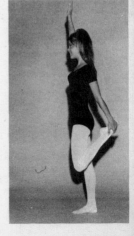

Fig. 174 (Right) Shift your full weight to your right leg. Bend your left knee and carefully bring your left foot up until you can hold it with your left hand. If you lose your balance, stop all movement and begin again. *Do not laugh at yourself.* Simply stop, compose yourself, and begin again.

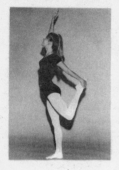

Fig. 175 (Left) The completed posture. The leg has been drawn upward as far as possible; the arm and head are brought back to aid in an intensive stretch of the spine. Stand as lightly as possible with your right leg. The lighter you make yourself feel, the easier it will be to maintain your balance. Hold for a count of five in the beginning and then ten when you have mastered the position.

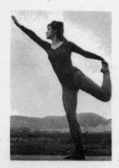

Fig. 176 This is a variation and a more advanced posture. When the count of Fig. 175 is completed, push back with your left foot and lower your right arm as illustrated. Hold as steady as possible for a count of five.

Lower your arm to the side and your foot to the floor and perform the identical movements with the left arm and right foot.

Alternate the sides and perform the Balance Posture routine three times.

176

BALANCE POSTURE

• Practice to attain smoothness in the movements.

> • Your balance will undoubtedly be shaky in the beginning, but this will pass quickly with practice.

• Never laugh at yourself or become discouraged if you lose your balance. This is not an easy exercise. Keep a serious attitude and you will accelerate your progress.

> • On some days this exercise will go more smoothly than on others. This is natural in the Yoga learning process.

• Remember that having control of your balance will make a pronounced difference in the way you look and feel. This exercise is well worth your dedicated effort.

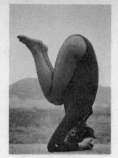

COMPLETED HEAD STAND

This is an advanced exercise in balance. The movements depicted below follow those of Fig. 7 of the Modified Head Stand on page 21.

Fig. 177 Now push against the floor with your toes and raise your legs very slowly and carefully to the position illustrated. Note that the back is held straight. It may require some weeks or even months to perfect this posture, but do not go farther until you feel completely secure in it. If you are shaky, simply hold this position for several moments and then return your feet to the floor. One or two more attempts will be sufficient for any given day. This is the way the body learns.

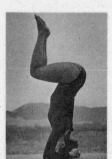

Fig. 178 (Center) Very slowly and carefully extend your legs upward. Again, you must feel that you have control of the movement.

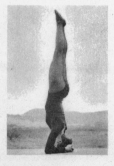

Fig. 179 (Bottom) The Completed Head Stand. Hold the posture as long as no discomfort is experienced.

178

Fig. 180 It is necessary to return your legs to the floor smoothly. Do not allow your feet to come crashing down. Bend your knees and begin slowly to lower your legs.

Fig. 181 (Center) Bring your knees farther down and in.

Fig. 182 (Below) Return your feet lightly to the floor. Keep your head and arms on the floor and rest in this position for at least thirty seconds. (You must not feel dizzy when you raise your head.)

Perform the Completed Head Stand once and hold whatever extreme position you attain for a comfortable period of time. Advanced students hold the completed posture for three to five minutes. A clock can be placed in a convenient position.

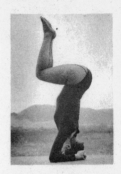

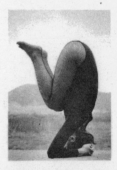

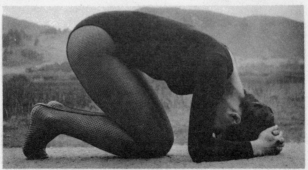

COMPLETED HEAD STAND

• All of the points listed under the Modified Head Stand apply also to this completed posture. You should reread them now

   • The benefits that the Modified Head Stand have for the face, scalp, hair, vision, hearing, etc., are increased with this completed posture. In addition, the Completed Head Stand has a wonderful effect on the brain's activity. Bringing an increased flow of blood into the head seems to refresh your brain, especially after the day's work. Advanced Yoga students are well aware of the truth of this statement.

• The main objective is, of course, to work for balance. This is a highly individual matter and must be left to the student's discretion. It is important not to become impatient in attempting to reach the extreme position. If you are not secure in Fig. 177 you should not attempt to go on. You must have control in each of the movements, otherwise you cannot expect to benefit fully and the great value of true balance will be lost.

• Some students use the wall as an aid during their initial practice. The body is placed close to the wall and it supports the back and legs in Figs. 177–79. However, you should not resort to the wall until you have attempted the movements many times and are convinced that no progress is being made.

• Surround yourself with a few pillows for added protection in the event that you lose your balance. Remember the suggestion that you place a small pillow or folded towel beneath your head before beginning.

• Thousands of Yoga students in their forties, fifties, and beyond, who, in their entire lives had never inverted their bodies, have accomplished the Completed Head Stand with sustained practice and patience.

CHAPTER 13

BEAUTY FOR THE INNER WOMAN

Unnatural *Glamour*	Natural *Beauty*
None.	Techniques to promote emotional stability, serenity, tranquility, vitality, enthusiasm, optimism, confidence, inner strength, harmony, elevation of consciousness, peace.

In applying the Yoga exercises to various areas of the body such as the face, waistline, legs, etc., we have been dealing with aspects of beauty that are quite tangible. We should now give our attention to some of its most important *abstract* qualities.

The vibrations of serenity, tranquility, and emotional stability are felt in the presence of a genuinely beautiful woman. She also imparts a sense of quiet vitality, and one has the impression that she is satisfied, fulfilled, and optimistic. Indeed, all of these qualities are synonymous with beauty. A woman subject to irritability, despondency, anger, envy, or various outbursts may be attractive, pretty, or glamorous but never beautiful.

The female is in harmony with herself—and able to transmit these harmonious vibrations to others—as a result of having found her self, her inner center. She has experienced some degree of self-realization. The Yoga exercises are designed to establish contact with this center and will certainly promote a feeling of great serenity. Because of their calming properties these exercises actually comprise a form of *meditation in movement*. In addition to the physical postures we have been doing, there are certain techniques, including those that make use of the breath, that deal in a very direct way with the mind and emotions.

Five Techniques for Inner Beauty

Five of these follow. The first three increase the supply of life-force and fill the organism with a certain confidence and vitality that is difficult to describe but will be quickly experienced. This is not nervous energy but a quiet strength and optimism. The fourth, Alternate Nostril Breathing, has the remarkable ability to soothe and stabilize the emotions, particularly after an upsetting experience. The final technique, Deep Relaxation, is the finest natural method to tranquilize, heal, and elevate the consciousness.

Women who are experiencing emotional problems, including those of personal relationships, should emphasize this section of exercises. The breathing practice often affords the opportunity to gain an objectivity or improved perspective of what is really involved in the problem at hand. Difficulties that seemingly have no resolution can simply dissolve when the consciousness is elevated.

People who need added strength to cope with negative habits can find it through these very exercises. Additional life-force supplied through the Complete and Charging Breaths has diminished or eliminated the need for smoking, alcohol, and drugs, as well as the cravings for harmful foods.

Women who are easily worried, upset, or depressed may find great relief through Alternate Nostril Breathing and Deep Relaxation. Again, when the life-force is increased, the emotions are quieted and stabilized and the illusionary nature of one's worries is often clearly seen. Remember that the birthright of every woman is to be fulfilled but that this can only be accomplished by learning how to turn inward and discover the self. The exercises of this section take you on just such a journey. Nowhere can the help and beauty of Yoga be experienced more directly than here.

COMPLETE BREATH—FOR VITALITY

The objective of this exercise is to fill the lungs completely. The usual "deep breathing" that is done in calisthenics will not accomplish the "complete breathing" of Yoga. To fill the lungs truly we must make three sets of movements *in conjunction with our inhalation*. This is really a breathing exercise of three stages that are explained below. Read the instructions through in their entirety before beginning.

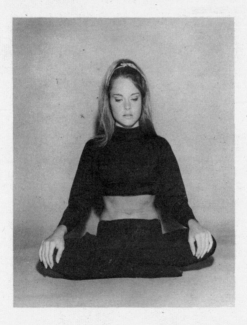

Fig. 183 Sit in a cross-legged posture. The Half-Lotus is best. First we want to empty our lungs completely. Therefore begin to exhale slowly through your nose. Pull your abdomen in as far as possible to aid in expelling the air from your lower lungs.

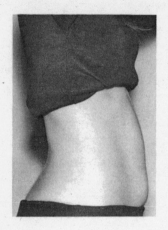 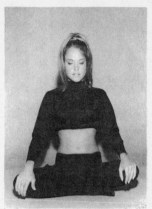

Fig. 184 (Left) Begin to inhale through your nose as slowly as possible. This inhalation is done so quietly and slowly that you can barely feel the air entering your nostrils. As you begin the inhalation you must *simultaneously* push down with your diaphragm and slowly distend your abdomen as far out as possible. This is accomplished with the use of the abdominal muscles. If this pushing out movement seems difficult, simply breathe normally and concentrate on practicing the slow distending of the abdomen.

This is the *first* part of the Complete Breath and should require approximately five seconds to execute.

Fig. 185 (Right) Continue to inhale slowly and quietly. Simultaneously pull your abdomen in and expand your chest as far as possible. Attempt to be conscious of your ribs and to feel that they also expand. The more exaggerated you can make this expansion of your entire chest area, the more your lungs will be filled.

This is the *second* part of the Complete Breath and should also require approximately five seconds.

Fig. 186 The final position. Continue the inhalation and slowly raise your shoulders as high as possible. Your body need not be held tensed. This movement should require the final five seconds, making fifteen seconds for the entire inhalation. Thus, once you learn the movements, you will be counting fifteen to complete the inhalation.

Retain your breath for a count of five.

Very slowly exhale through your nose and empty your lungs during a count of fifteen. There are no special physical movements required during the exhalation; the body simply relaxes. At the count of fifteen you should have drawn in your abdomen, completely emptied your lungs, and gone back to the position of Fig. 183. Without pause, begin the next count of fifteen and repeat.

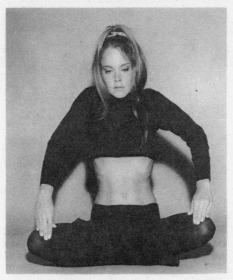

Summary: *Inhalation*

Abdominal movements	5 seconds
Chest expansion	5 seconds
Shoulder movements	5 seconds
Retention of breath	5 seconds
Exhalation and relaxation of body	15 seconds

Perform the Complete Breath routine five times.

COMPLETE BREATH

• Although this exercise is given in three parts, once it is learned, the movements should flow into one another so that there is no break.

> • The first movement, where the abdomen is distended, usually requires practice to perfect, especially since we are simultaneously *inhaling*. We are usually taught to *pull the abdomen in* during a deep breath. However, this actually inhibits the air from filling the lower part of the lungs, hence our distending the abdomen rather than pulling in. There is nothing "natural" about contracting the abdomen during an inhalation. It is an erroneous habit that can be unlearned.

• Your body need never become tense or rigid during the movements.

> • Most advanced students lower (not close) the eyelids when performing the Complete Breath. This aids in concentration on the breathing.

• The Complete Breath can be done almost anywhere when you need to clear your mind and revitalize. You can do it while walking, sitting in a bus, car, airplane (it is one of the best of all techniques to overcome motionsickness and nausea), before an important meeting, during a tense situation, etc. When performing the Complete Breath in such circumstances or while in the presence of other persons, do not raise the shoulders. In this way you can do the movements without calling attention to yourself.

> • This is an excellent breathing exercise to help negate some of the deadly effects of cigarette smoking and air pollution.

• Keep in mind the main point of the Complete Breath: The condition of your blood (which constantly affects every aspect of your existence) is largely dependent on the amount and quality of air you are breathing. The more "completely" you are able to breathe, the more "alive" you are going to feel and the more vitality and beauty you will radiate.

COMPLETE BREATH (STANDING)—
FOR VITALITY

We are able to fill the lungs still further and experience an even greater revitalization if we perform the Complete Breath in conjunction with the standing movements outlined below.

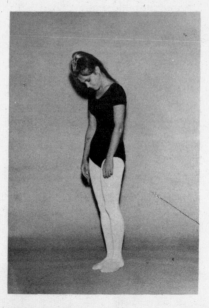

Fig. 187 Stand directly on the floor, not on the mat. Your feet are close together. Begin the deep exhalation of the Complete Breath. Simultaneously pull your abdomen in and allow your trunk to become limp as illustrated.

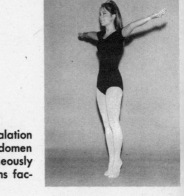

Fig. 188 Begin the deep inhalation and slowly expand your abdomen as previously learned. Simultaneously begin to raise your arms, palms facing upward.

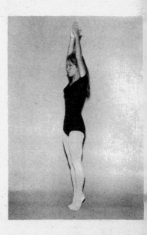

Fig. 189 Continue the deep inhalation. Contract your abdomen and expand your chest. Simultaneously rise on your toes and bring your palms to touch overhead. Note that your elbows are straight. Hold this position and retain the breath for a count of five.

Begin the deep exhalation. Simultaneously lower the soles of your feet to the floor and bring your arms back to your sides. Continue to exhale and return to the position of Fig. 187.

Without pause begin the deep exhalation and repeat.

Perform the Complete Breath (Standing) three to five times.

CHARGING BREATH—FOR VITALITY

In this second breathing exercise we use the air to "charge" ourselves in much the same way as a battery is charged from a generator. The "generator" in this case is the air, and with the following technique we can increase our energy and vitality by quickly extracting life-force.

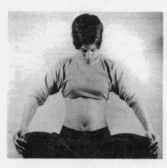

Fig. 190 Sit in a cross-legged posture. There are only two movements in this exercise: an inhalation accompanied by an expansion of the abdomen and an exhalation accompanied by a contraction of the abdomen. These movements are performed *quickly, forcefully, and rhythmically.* Inhale through your nose and simultaneously expand your abdomen. This movement is identical with the first part of the Complete Breath.

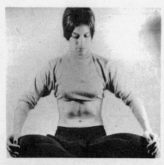

Fig. 191 Without pause, quickly contract your abdomen as forcefully as possible. Simultaneously exhale through your nose. If you do this contracting movement with sufficient force you will empty your lungs. Without pause, begin the next inhalation and expand your abdomen. Repeat these movements quickly but rhythmically so that you can eventually do a series of fifteen in about seven seconds.

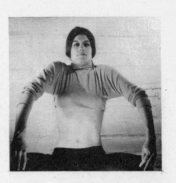

Fig. 192 Immediately following the fifteenth Charging Breath, perform the Complete Breath. Retain the air as we have done previously in the Complete Breath.

Fig. 193 Now, during the retention, *tap your chest very forcefully with your middle finger.* This is a hammer-like movement (similar to that used by a physician when listening to the lungs) that begins at the top of your chest and works fairly rapidly across and back, down to your abdomen. You will have to retain the air for approximately ten seconds to tap forcefully throughout the chest. This movement stimulates your lung cells. Place your hand back on your knee and slowly exhale.

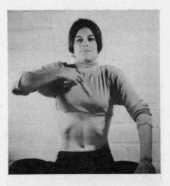

Perform the entire routine of the Charging Breath, which includes the series of fifteen breaths and the Complete Breath with tapping, five times.

ALTERNATE NOSTRIL BREATHING— FOR EMOTIONAL STABILITY

Our third and final breathing exercise is done in four parts: inhalation, retention, exhalation, suspension. These are applied to the flow of the breath as follows:

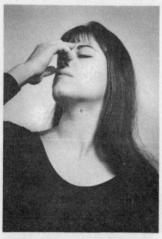

Fig. 194 Sit in a cross-legged posture. Place your right hand in the position depicted. Your right thumb is adjacent to your right nostril, your ring finger is adjacent to your left nostril, your index and middle fingers are together between your eyebrows. Your hand is relaxed and your eyelids are lowered (not closed).

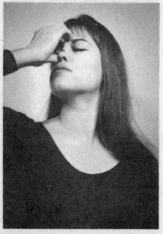

Fig. 195 Execute a deep exhalation through both nostrils. Gently press your *right* nostril closed with your thumb and slowly inhale a quiet, deep breath through your *left* nostril. The first two movements of the Complete Breath, the expanding of your abdomen and chest, are performed during this inhalation. The third movement of the Complete Breath, the raising of your shoulders, is not done.

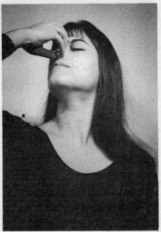

Fig. 196 When the inhalation is completed press your *left* nostril closed with your ring finger. Both nostrils are now closed and the air is retained.

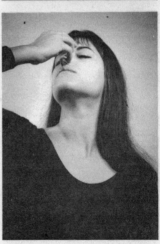

Fig. 197 Your left nostril remains closed but your *right* nostril is now opened. Slowly and quietly exhale deeply through your *right* nostril.

When the exhalation is completed, close your *right* nostril. Both nostrils are now closed, your lungs are empty, and breathing is suspended.

Now repeat the identical routine, but this time reverse the flow of the air in your nostrils. That is, hold your *left* nostril closed, open your *right* nostril (the exhalation has just occurred through the right nostril), and inhale as before. Keep your hand relaxed and your eyelids lowered. Do not allow your trunk to slump.

When the inhalation is completed, press the *right* nostril closed (both nostrils are now closed) and retain.

Open the *left* nostril (the right remains closed) and exhale deeply.

Close both nostrils and suspend.

This completes *one round,* since we have returned to the original starting point.

Without pause, reverse the flow of the breath once again and begin the second round: open the *left* nostril and inhale, etc.

We derive the greatest benefits, in terms of quieting and strengthening the emotions, when we execute these breathing movements in a strict, precise rhythm. The rhythm we will use is as follows: inhale—eight beats, retain—four beats, exhale—eight beats, suspend—four beats, inhale—eight beats, etc. Therefore, as you begin your Alternate Nostril Breathing, start the beat in your mind and keep it going as a metronome. It is essential that the rhythm be absolutely steady. Some students find that tapping the floor lightly with the index finger of the left hand aids in maintaining the strict rhythm.

Summary:	Inhale through the left	8 beats
	Retain (both nostrils closed)	4 beats
	Exhale through the right	8 beats
	Suspend (both nostrils closed)	4 beats
	Inhale through the right	8 beats
	Retain (both nostrils closed)	4 beats
	Exhale through the left	8 beats
	Suspend (both nostrils closed)	4 beats

THIS COMPLETES ONE ROUND

Perform five rounds of Alternate Nostril Breathing.

When you have completed the final round, place your right hand on your knee and remain absolutely still for two to three minutes. You will experience a rare feeling of stability and peacefulness.

DEEP RELAXATION—FOR TRANQUILITY

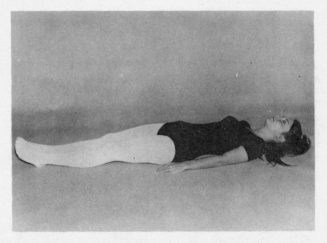

Fig. 198 (Above) Lie with your back and head on the mat. Close your eyes. Become aware of the various parts of your body, your face, neck, arms, shoulders, legs, feet, etc., and allow each to adjust itself to its most comfortable position. All muscles relax. Nothing is held tensed.

Next, attempt to empty your mind of all present thoughts. Maintain your mind quietly so that no thoughts will arise for the next several minutes. It will be necessary to focus your full attention on a visual image.

Fig. 199 (Below) When a state of deep quietude has been reached by following the above directions, place your fingertips on your solar plexus as illustrated.

Begin a slow inhalation. This is not the Complete Breath, and we will perform no extra physical movements other than those necessary during an inhalation.

During the inhalation attempt to visualize in your mind's eye a very intense white light which is being drawn from your solar plexus into your fingertips. Try to visualize this white light as being more brilliant than sunlight, similar to that of an X ray.

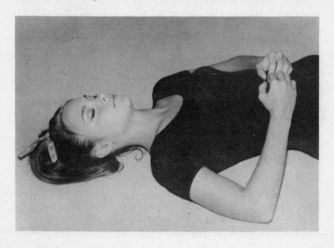

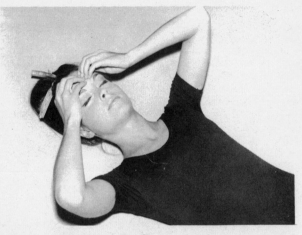

Fig. 200 When the inhalation is completed, retain the air and transfer your fingertips to rest between your eyebrows.

Begin to exhale slowly. During the exhalation, attempt to visualize the white light flowing from your fingertips into your head. The entire area surrounding your head is bathed in a brilliant illumination. When the exhalation is completed, return your fingertips to your solar plexus and repeat.

Perform seven rounds of the Deep Relaxation technique.

DEEP RELAXATION

• This technique has been used for countless centuries to elevate the level of consciousness. It also has healing properties and can be utilized to aid in the relief of pain, discomfort, and illness. When used for the latter, the inhalation is the same as described above but during the exhalation the fingertips are placed on the troubled area. The white light is then visualized as flowing into and illuminating the area in question. Deep Relaxation may be performed in a cross-legged posture if the hands need to be moved to an area of the back or legs.

• Some students have difficulty in visualizing the white light; either they cannot see it at all or it appears and fades. To visualize continually requires intensive concentration, what in Yoga is known as "one-pointedness." For this you must practice. Practicing to achieve one-pointedness will be of great value to you, not only in Yoga, but in all of your daily activities.

• If you find that it is absolutely impossible for you to visualize the white light, simply place your full attention on the breathing and allow nothing to distract you.

- It is essential to keep your mind clear; consequently you must be alert to any thoughts that begin to arise. Gently banish such thoughts and return your attention to the visualization.

- The results of Deep Relaxation cannot be described. They can only be experienced.

CHAPTER
14

PRACTICE PLAN

The following Practice Plan is suggested to permit you to exercise, in a minimum of time, all areas of the body on each day of practice.

The exercises in this book are included in the three groups below. Each group represents a possible practice routine for one day. The routines are arranged so that all exercises will be performed in the course of three days. These groups should be continually rotated.

In the event you are working on a particular problem area of your body, you should stress *all of the exercises in that category each time you practice*. For example, if you are attempting to reduce inches in the waistline, you should perform the five exercises listed under Beauty for the Waistline each day. In the charts below these five exercises are divided among three days.

These charts are suggestions only. You may wish to devise a practice plan more suitable for your particular needs.

Remember that exercises such as the Cobra, Complete Breath, Alternate Nostril Breathing, and others have been suggested for use whenever needed. If you were to utilize one or more of these at some point during the day you would nonetheless include them in your practice time if the routine of that day so indicated.

Practice during menstruation—This varies widely among students. Some are unable to do any exercising whatsoever, others find that discomfort of the period has been greatly reduced through practice of the milder stretching, breathing, and inverted positions. You will have to experiment to determine what is best for you.

Practice during pregnancy—It is essential to consult your physician regarding the activities you may undertake during pregnancy. The majority of my students have continued all of the exercises during the first four to five months. In the later stages many have continued the milder stretching postures. The breathing exercises, especially the Complete Breath and the Alternate Nostril Breathing, can be performed throughout pregnancy, and these are very similar to certain of the breathing techniques taught in natural childbirth.

The firming and strengthening postures such as the Abdominal Lifts, Lotus, Side Raise, Back Push-up, and Slow-motion Firming, as well as the inverted positions, such as in the Plough, Shoulder Stand, and Head Stand, have proven extremely valuable in the postnatal period.

Practice during menopause—It has been the experience of my students that there is no better natural practice than that of Yoga to minimize the physical as well as the emotional and mental disturbances that often occur during the menopause. All of the Yoga exercises outlined in this book should be seriously practiced with increased emphasis on those presented in the Beauty for the Inner Woman section.

(Refer to the directions
of each exercise for com-
plete information regarding
timing and repetition.)

1

HAIR	Scalp Exercise
FACE	Modified Head Stand
CHIN	Chin Exercise
NECK	Head Roll
BUST	Chest Expansion Hand Clasp
ABDOMEN	Abdominal Lifts: Standing All Fours Seated
BACK	Cobra
HIPS AND THIGHS	Side Bend
WAISTLINE	Circular Motion
LEGS	Leg Clasp
FEET AND ANKLES	Backward Bend
BALANCE AND POISE	Toe Twist
REGENERA-TION	Complete Breath Complete Breath (Standing)

2	3
Scalp Exercise	Scalp Exercise
Lion	Lion
Chin Exercise	Chin Exercise
Head Twist	Head Roll
Bust Exercise	Bow
Locust	Slow-motion Firming
Back Stretch Plough	Twist
Leg Raise	Back Push-up Leg Over
Triangle Shoulder Stand	Standing Twist Elbow-to-Knee
Knee and Thigh Stretch	Alternate Leg Pull
Backward Bend	Backward Bend
Balance Posture	Completed Head Stand
Charging Breath	Alternate Nostril Breathing

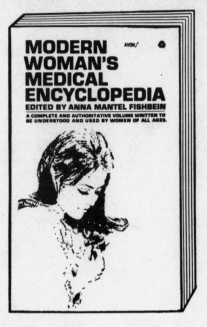